PRAISE FOR

Rhonda Britten

"You've seen her as life coach on the Emmy Award–winning *Starting Over*. Now start over yourself with advice on accepting your body type."

—*Library Journal*

"Rhonda Britten has risen from the ashes of genuine catastrophe . . . What she has accomplished . . . and now helps others to accomplish as well, is nothing short of miraculous.

—Marianne Williamson,
New York Times bestselling author
of *A Return to Love* and *Illuminata*

"Rhonda Britten can show you how to leave your fear behind and live your life with freedom and joy."

—Dave Pelzer,
New York Times bestselling author
of *A Child Called "It"* and *A Man Named Dave*

"Ms. Britten gives the reader thoughtful and creative approaches to conquering fear and doubt in order to love unencumbered."

—Dr. Fred Luskin,
director of the Stanford University Forgiveness Project,
author of *Forgive for Good*

Do I Look Fat in This?

Get Over Your Body

and On With Your Life

RHONDA BRITTEN

A PERIGEE BOOK

A PERIGEE BOOK
Published by Penguin Group
Penguin Group (USA) Inc.
375 Hudson Street, New York, New York 10014, USA

Penguin Group (Canada), 90 Eglinton Avenue East, Suite 700, Toronto, Ontario M4P 2Y3,
Canada (a division of Pearson Penguin Canada Inc.)
Penguin Books Ltd., 80 Strand, London WC2R 0RL, England
Penguin Ireland, 25 St. Stephen's Green, Dublin 2, Ireland (a division of Penguin Books Ltd.)
Penguin Group (Australia), 250 Camberwell Road, Camberwell, Victoria 3124, Australia
(a division of Pearson Australia Group Pty. Ltd.)
Penguin Books India Pvt. Ltd., 11 Community Centre, Panchsheel Park, New Delhi—110 017, India
Penguin Group (NZ), 67 Apollo Drive, Mairangi Bay, Auckland 1311, New Zealand
(a division of Pearson New Zealand Ltd.)
Penguin Books (South Africa) (Pty.) Ltd., 24 Sturdee Avenue, Rosebank, Johannesburg 2196,
South Africa

Penguin Books Ltd., Registered Offices: 80 Strand, London WC2R 0RL, England

While the author has made every effort to provide accurate telephone numbers and Internet addresses
at the time of publication, neither the publisher nor the author assumes any responsibility for errors, or
for changes that occur after publication. Further, the publisher does not have any control over and does
not assume any responsibility for author or third-party websites or their content.

PRINTING HISTORY
G. P. Putnam's Sons hardcover edition / February 2006
Perigee trade paperback edition / March 2007

Perigee trade paperback ISBN: 978-0-399-53312-9

The Library of Congress has cataloged the G. P. Putnam's Sons hardcover edition as follows:

Britten, Rhonda.
    Do I look fat in this? : get over your body and on with your life /
by Rhonda Britten.—1st ed.
        p. cm.
    ISBN 0-525-94945-3 (hardcover)
    1. Body image in women.   2. Women—Psychology.   I. Title.
    BF697.5.B63B75   2006
    306.4'613—dc22   2005034236

PRINTED IN THE UNITED STATES OF AMERICA

10 9 8 7 6 5 4 3 2 1

Most Perigee Books are available at special quantity discounts for bulk purchases for sales promo-
tions, premiums, fund-raising, or educational use. Special books, or book excerpts, can also be created
to fit specific needs. For details, write: Special Markets, The Berkley Publishing Group, 375 Hudson
Street, New York, New York 10014.

Dedicated to my dear friend Marta, who forced me to face my body when it was the last thing I wanted to do.

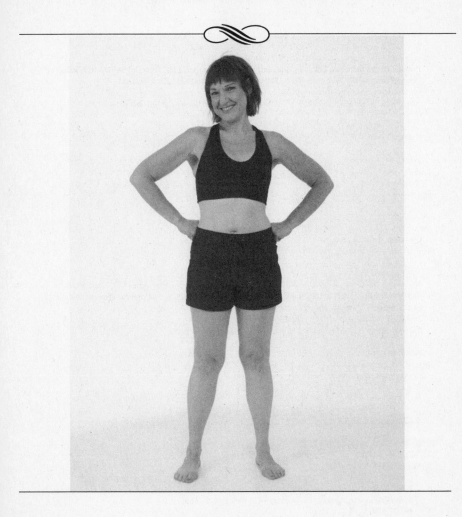

MARTA

After 40-pound Weight Loss

Height: 5' 4½" • Weight: 139 pounds • Age: 53

Body Image: *I love my body more than I ever have!*

CONTENTS

CONTENTS

LETTER TO THE READER

After writing three previously published and best-selling books, I consider myself to be a somewhat courageous writer—someone unafraid of going deep and baring her soul. If I thought that what I had gone through could help others, I had little hesitancy in exposing it. Within the pages of each of my books, I shared many personal things—including my parents' horrific death at the hand of my father, my painful divorce from a man I was deeply in love with, and my insecurities as a woman in her forties in the intimidating world of dating. I wrote about my ups and downs, and everything in between. But in spite of all that self-revealing, this time around, that experience and confidence has been useless in writing the book you now hold in your hands. Sharing how I feel about my body and my body image—putting it all into words on paper for you to read—has brought every one of my vulnerabilities to the surface. This, by far, is my most difficult book to date.

When I began writing *Fearless Living*, my first book, I was an inexperienced writer, but the subject matter was something I knew well. I had taught various forms of Fearless Living in workshops and seminars for years, and had seen the strength of the information. I knew the principles I was espousing had also transformed my life, so in the midst of my unschooled writing, I had faith that the book was, in and of itself, valuable and important. I believed it would change people's lives. I was sharing what I knew, after the fact—after I had honed the tools for myself. Sure, I was scared; it was my first book. But the vulnerable parts of myself that I was sharing, I had already healed. I had already grieved for and forgiven my parents' deaths. I had already moved past my divorce. I had already uncovered the mechanics of fear. I was writing from a historical perspective.

My next book, *Fearless Loving*, felt equally important, but with one successful book under my belt, I felt even safer sharing my journey through love. Heck, hadn't I helped countless men and women find love? I knew that what I was writing about worked. Single women by the hundreds took my workshops, and soon, reports were coming in that more and more of them were hearing wedding bells. I had practiced the dating principles myself for years, with loving results. Everyone said they felt more love in their lives after incorporating the tools I shared. All I had to do was write down what I knew. This, too, was a book based largely in the past.

Change Your Life in 30 Days, my third book, was the easiest to write. Based on my workshops and speaking events, I knew what people wanted. I chronicled the journey of transformation I had taught from the beginning of my life-coaching practice ten years ago, and included all the topics I regularly discussed, all the tools and skills I'd assigned to hundreds of my clients and the proven principles of change, but had never written down, all of the things my clients and workshop attendees seemed to clamor to hear and wanted me to repeat over and over again. I completed the book in less than thirty days.

The book you now hold in your hands, however, has been a completely different experience for me—and one that I'm not entirely comfortable with yet. I have been working in earnest on my body image for the past three years. This issue is on the surface of every aspect of my life, and I have learned so much. I have learned that you can't hide from your body, no matter how hard you try. I have learned that you can deny your fears for years, or avoid love for decades, but that's not so easy when it comes to your body. We use our bodies every day. They're front and center—going with us wherever we go. Your body, my body, is right out there for all the world to see.

At this moment, I am sitting at my favorite restaurant in Los Angeles—a busy, bustling, yet cozy place called Marmalade Café. The managers have become friends, and no one seems to mind that I often sit for hours at my table typing away. As always, I have ordered an egg-white frittata, chock-full of vegetables, with a side of French toast, covered in blueberries, bananas, strawberries, and maple syrup. Healthy to some, indulgent to others. While my feast is being delivered to my table, the woman next to me leans over and asks me if I am an author. "Yes!" I answer with pride. Having fantasized about being a writer for most of my life, now that I am, it is not only a goal accomplished, but more importantly, a dream fulfilled.

"What are you writing about?" the woman asks hesitantly.

"Body image," I blurt out, noticing how almost immediately she begins to eye me with suspicion. Actually, as the woman speaks to me about how she thinks that sounds interesting, and blah, blah, blah, she is totally checking out my body! It's not even like she's trying to pretend otherwise, as her eyes deliberately scan my form from head to toe, landing for an uncomfortably long moment on my outwardly stretched belly.

I know what she's thinking. I swear I can hear her inner chatter. *You? Writing a book on body image? You don't have that great of a body. I sure wouldn't want to read anything you have to say, if the goal is to look like you.*

And on it goes . . .

And French toast? You shouldn't be eating all that bread and sugar if you care about your body. What kind of expert could you be?!

"My salad is absolutely delicious," she announces, interrupting my thoughts. *Is that a hint?* I wonder. I pull my sweater closer.

This woman would be hard-pressed to knock me for being the author of my past three books. I mean, who can argue that I know a thing or two about fear? I've lived through some of the worst experiences life can dish out. But, to write as an expert on the body? Well, you just have to look at mine to easily surmise that I probably don't have much worth saying.

Ironically, to some people, I will be seen as too thin (and have always been too thin, despite being fat for *me*) to know the pain of being truly fat, and therefore, I will never understand what it is like to be overweight. While to others, particularly people who admire the supermodel ideal, I will be seen as too chunky to be taken seriously. Everyone will have an opinion. That is frightening, to say the least.

It is bad enough that I already judge my body so harshly. Although I've been healing in leaps and bounds from where I was three years ago, or even six months ago, my body image is still fragile. I work on loving it, and myself, every day, but I am not yet free from feeling bad about what still jiggles or squishes on my body. I am not totally out of the woods. Negative thoughts still creep in to ruin my day, although thankfully with much less regularity. Perhaps this sounds familiar. Perhaps you know the feeling.

Even though writing a book about body image is the scariest

thing I have ever done (and makes this fear expert feel mighty fearful), I don't know what else to do but to put myself out there. I decided long ago that my life would be about turning pain into empowerment. So, here goes. I pray that I will have the courage to handle any judgments or criticisms that come my way.

This feeling of vulnerability is where I write from. This is where I am, as I share what I know (and am learning) about a topic that I am still working through myself. My body is something that is alive and breathing, and it's a joy to be embracing it more and more. But I have yet to be healed from this perilous journey of body transformation, yet I can see and feel enough success to keep me going. I now love my body and myself more than not. I have conquered many of my body limitations (amazed by the things I can now do, things that I previously thought were only reserved for "athletes"), and have let go of much of my negative self-talk. I am better than ever, inside and out.

I humbly offer this book as a testament of one woman's journey. A woman who feels fat some days and thin on those very rare occasions. A woman who is doing her best to face her inner demons of body madness and come from a healed and happy perspective, regardless of how I look—whether it's a "good" or "bad" body day. A woman who has learned something she never thought possible: *that her body can be her very best friend.*

Do I Look Fat
in This?

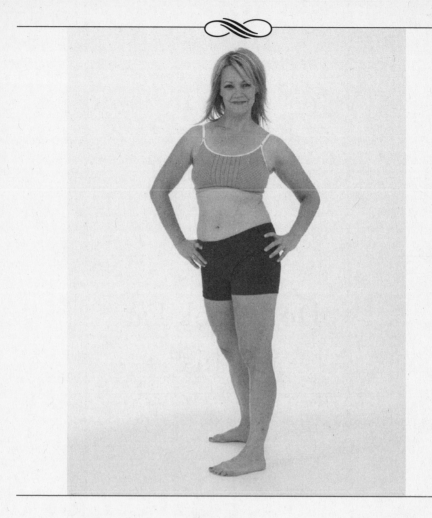

RHONDA

Height: 5'5½" • Weight: 142 pounds • Age: 45

Body Philosophy: *My body is my partner and only together can we create a life filled with health, happiness, and love.*

Why Me? Why Now?

Arriving in Los Angeles, the city of glamorous angels, was overwhelming for me—a girl who grew up in the Midwest. There were so many beautiful people, seemingly everywhere I went. I had driven across the country, convinced that moving was the answer, and that I would make it as an actress. But at my auditions, I was never up for the lead role; instead I always read for the part of the sister of the star or the best friend of the cousin twice removed. One thing became clear, even though no one stated it out loud: *I wasn't thin enough to be at the front of the line*. Even at my thinnest, at the age of twenty-five, I still felt like a giant compared to the other actresses in the room. I figured I was a good twenty pounds from getting the roles I wanted. You learn fast in Hollywood that your weight, not necessarily your talent, often determines the parts you play. I wasn't even in the same universe as the leading ladies I longed to be.

Living in Los Angeles forced me to face the insecurities that had brought me to leave my home state of Minnesota in the first place. I had always wanted more for my life. Aching to leave behind a terrifying childhood, I assumed that everything would start anew in the land of sun and fun. In my plans, the Golden State would envelop me in its shining goodness, delivering me fame and fortune. I had it all mapped out. Like so many people before, I looked to this place of opportunity to lighten my load and brighten my life.

No one thought to tell me that in leaving your problems behind, they miss you and come racing out after you (sort of like the cat whose humans move, only to find that the mangy-looking feline on the porch just risked life and limb to walk two thousand miles to the new house). After a few months in my new hometown, my prior eight lives showed up with a vengeance, and there was no denying that much to my chagrin, I was still the same ol' Rhonda Britten I had always been . . . the girl who hadn't been smart enough or worthy enough to save her parents' lives. The girl who probably didn't even deserve to live herself. Needless to say, I had some inner work to do. After some hard knocks, I understood that it was essential that I figure out how to heal my past. That was a long and arduous process—one I explain in depth in *Fearless Living*, and highlight briefly in the coming pages. As I made the transition from a woman out of control (in other words, attempting to carry out my own suicide) to one who was living on integrity and increasing amounts of self-love, acting no longer interested me. I got tired of reading lines about fictitious characters who led better lives than I did. I was sick of pretending to be someone else night after night, play after play.

I realized that it was easy for me to act, but extremely hard for me to be myself. Acting gave me an escape—something I had needed for years—but no longer wanted. I knew that the only way to find out who I was, was to practice being myself, rather than using my finite time and energy learning how to become somebody else. I didn't want to *be* the entertainment; I wanted to be entertained by my own thoughts, my own wisdom, and my own company. So I quit. No notice. No good-byes. I just left my agent and walked away from a lifelong dream that had been borne from my need to feel special.

How ironic that I am now the Life Coach on an Emmy Award–winning daytime reality show *Starting Over*. Not as an actress, but as myself. Five days a week for years now, I've appeared on television—something that, when I was younger, was one of the ultimate things a person could accomplish. But today, rather than playing a role on a series, I get to be authentic. Real. *Me!* Someone actually wants me to be me, with no faking, no pretending, and no acting involved. Never in my wildest childhood imaginings could I have foreseen that I'd no longer have to act to be accepted. This, to me, validates all of my hard work. It validates that when you are true to yourself, good things happen. I count this amongst the greatest victories of my life. That I can be myself, and be accepted for it.

Or can I?

The message board on Startingovertv.com is a gathering place for the fans of *Starting Over*. Some of those fans love me; others despise me. Some don't seem to feel one way or the other, but use me as a mere topic of conversation. When I signed on to do the show, I thought it would be different for me than for other television personalities, and I wouldn't be an object of intense scrutiny. After all, I don't date famous movie stars or walk around with an entourage. I don't spend $2,000 on a sequin-studded jacket for my dog. I change lives, including my own. I thought that's what the message boards were for—spreading healing through community—and it would be the healing that viewers would tune in for and comment on. My coaching skills, the exercises I create, and the transformations . . .

that would be the focus, right? But I quickly and painfully learned that it doesn't matter if you are an actress or a Life Coach. If your mug makes it into Jane Doe's living room, you are fair game.

My initiation came within weeks of the first episode. . . .

"Is Rhonda pregnant?" wrote Fan #1 in the heading of the message board. (I most certainly was not.) "Her stomach is huge. I hate those pants she had on," the text continued. "What was she thinking? Flowered pants on a pregnant woman just accentuate her growing bulge."

"I noticed that as well," replied Fan #2. "My bet is, yes. I think she was trying to cover it up with her top."

"And she looked really tired yesterday, too," continued the first. "Did you notice how baggy her eyes looked?"

I wanted to cry. What was I supposed to do, go under the knife and get an eye lift during all of my leisurely spare time? So someone else could post a message saying, *"Did you catch Rhonda's eye job? She looks so fake!"*

On and on these messages went, rambling about the don'ts of my appearance, as if these "fans" had suddenly been put in charge of the worst-dressed list of self-help TV. I sat there staring at the computer in disbelief. These particular fans could care less about my coaching. They only seemed to care about my looks!

I sat there for hours digesting what had just happened. I obsessively relived the day I wore those pants, trying to determine how I had felt about my looks. I had really thought I looked good. I had been having what I call a "thin day," otherwise I assure you that I would not have had the courage to wear those pants—not when skirts hide so much more.

You want reality? Here's the reality of my glitzy life as a reality television "star." I wake up each day two hours before I am supposed to arrive at the *Starting Over* house so I can do my own makeup and hair. I have no image consultant or stylist at my command. There is no one at the ready with brushes and gloss in hand for touch-ups. No one is combing or fluffing my hair, which is why you often see it flat as a pancake at the end of the day. I do it all. I am not a trained makeup artist or salon-trained hairstylist, but I will be judged as if I were. And my body will be judged no matter what I wear or how much weight I lose. I see that now. But that doesn't make it easy.

Do I look fat in this? is what I have asked myself every day since I was in junior high school. And since my first devastating experience on the message board, I realize that, even now, my life is run by my weight.

My friend Linda tells me that she is proud of me. I didn't wait to get thin before appearing on television. *"You could have delayed your dreams, stayed safely out of sight until the pounds came off . . . if they came off,"* she says. And that's true. I've come to acknowledge myself for putting myself in the ring, despite my insecurities. But it's one thing to look at your body in the mirror, and quite another to see it blown up on a screen so that every fat roll is accentuated, every wrinkle is magnified, and every physical weakness amplified. God forbid I miss a few hours of beauty sleep! They say the television adds ten pounds. It feels like twenty. But beyond weight, the camera threatens to shatter any trace of self-esteem I possess.

After my move to drive-or-perish Los Angeles, I rode my ten-speed bicycle everywhere. I partied every night at the clubs and danced my butt off. I worked during the day as a waitress, lifting heavy trays of food that kept my arms taut and toned. I was in killer shape (the best shape of my life), but I still worried about the size of my hips, the extra weight on the inside of my thighs, and whether my tummy was flat enough. While I did have men interested in me, I didn't believe they really cared about me as a person (I was too flawed to really be loved, after all). My body might have been at its best, but emotionally I was at my worst. I had no real friends to speak of or career opportunities. If I just had a better body, I reasoned, then my life would begin. But it never happened. Looking back, that was my best body to date and I sadly never enjoyed it.

And that has been the dilemma until now. As I faced my fears and got healthier emotionally, I packed on the pounds. I hit my highest weight after I quit acting and didn't have a clue who I was or what I should do next. And it has taken me years to face the shame that weight has induced. It took transforming other areas of my life before I ever had the courage to face my body issues—honestly, there were some mornings I didn't even know how to get out of bed, let alone jump on the treadmill or give up sugar.

This book is the story of how I went from disliking my body to celebrating it, from hating my hips to appreciating their beauty and function. More importantly, I'm learning to let go of perfection and finally accept who I am, including the number on the scale and the ticks on the measuring tape. Learning to face the fact that you are your body and at the same time, that you are more than your body, you will find the freedom you need to finally love all of you. Together, we will discover that body image does not have to control our lives or make our decisions for us. The past does not dictate the future. In the upcoming chapters, I've included exercises that I use with my private clients, as well as on *Starting Over,* and others I have created for myself. And yes, men will find benefits here too!

Getting over your body isn't about giving up. I want you to get on with your life and no longer allow your body to stop you from doing anything you are physically capable of doing. Because today, in the body I have, I do affect people, make a difference, and feel special in my own way. And isn't that what we all want? Your body isn't stopping you. You are. I want you to be happy in your own skin, and embracing a healthy body image is crucial for you to claim your life as your own.

I invite you to join me in transforming our bodies, and the way we look at them. Doing so will open your heart and change your life. I know. I'm living this daily, and I'm so excited to have you on board.

Let's begin. . . .

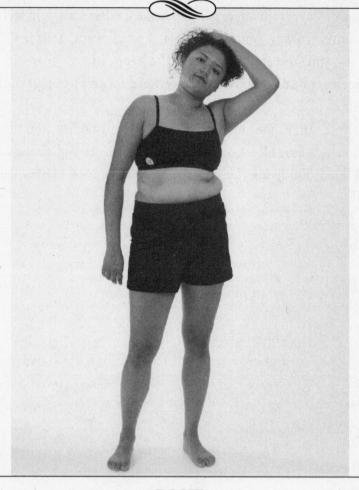

ROSIE

The Typical American Woman

Height: 5'5"   •   Weight: 154 pounds   •   Age: 23

Body Thoughts: *I love my legs and breasts but
hate my stomach and hips.*

CHAPTER 1

Why Do I Feel So Fat?

I have just finished speaking in front of a thousand people for the *Starting Over in America* mall tour. It's our tenth stop on the fifteen-city tour, and the surroundings are so similar to the other malls we've traveled to that I can barely remember what part of the country we're in. For the last two hours, I've been hugged and thanked by throngs of mostly women who are strangers to me, but who treat me like family. They wrap their arms around me and bare their souls. Some laugh. Many cry. All of them touch my heart. They patiently stand in line waiting for autographs, chatting and laughing amongst themselves, as if they're just excited to be in the same building as me, the *Starting Over* Life Coach.

Starting Over is a dramatic reality series that airs five days a week throughout the country. Its purpose: to change people's lives. At any one time, you can tune in to find six women living under one roof, battling their demons until they face their issues, do the hard work to resolve their problems, and achieve their dreams. As one woman completes her goal, another one takes her place. Each year we have approximately twenty-three graduates, with millions of viewers at home, pen and paper in hand, changing their lives right alongside the women on TV. I consider it a high honor to be the original Life Coach on a show that's been praised everywhere from *TV Guide* to the *New York Times*.

It's obvious by the faces standing before me that *Starting Over* has touched these women deeply and made a tangible difference in their lives. I tell myself that they'd feel this way about any coach who might be on the show, but it feels so personal. They shower me with the details of the impact *I've* made in their minds, habits, and hearts. They give me gifts and cards. I feel connected and loved. And they say just the words that I long to hear. Over and over my favorite compliments spill out of their mouths . . .

> *"Oh, you look so thin!"*
> *"You're so much smaller in person!"*
> *"Rhonda, you're so petite. You're tiny!"*
> *"You've saved my life. By the way, I love your hair. Where do you get it done?"*
> *"Thank you, Rhonda!"* come screams from the second floor balcony. *"We love you!"*

I'm thinking, *Wow. This is GREAT! I look great. I'm making a difference, and the fans tell me I'm thin. Life is good!* I feel so full of love. So confident. Suddenly, it doesn't matter that my stomach still pooches over my skirt, or that I can feel my thighs rubbing together as we speak. No one cares. It's not about the size of my pants (which are still larger than I'd like), because no one's perfect. It's about my ability to help change our viewers' lives, which seems to happen no matter what I weigh.

I feel so grateful. I had hoped, but had never quite known for sure until this moment, that my life could be this good.

The publicist tells me it's time to go. No more books to sign. We've got to keep to our schedule. I walk in the direction of our car as hundreds of women wave and clap and see me off.

Back at the hotel, I'm walking through the lobby feeling high on life. I pass by the reception area and see a cover of the latest fashion magazine with a gorgeous, skinny woman on the cover. Normally this would make me feel fat, but as I stop to look at her flawless image, I smile inside. I've been working hard on my body image, and today proves it. I accepted compliments. I actually felt good inside my body. I'm not going to compare myself to her. She's airbrushed anyway; everyone knows that. She's not *real*.

I get in the elevator to go to my room on the twentieth floor. On the third floor the elevator stops and the doors open. Who gets on the elevator with me but a five-ten, gorgeous, forty-plus-year-old woman who couldn't weigh more than 125 pounds! She looks like a walking, airbrushed, only slightly older replica of the cover I just saw. *My gosh, I'm getting it from both sides,* I think to myself. As we ride the next seventeen floors in silence, I wonder if there's some cosmic conspiracy out there trying to knock me off my pedestal, reminding me that I'm not so beautiful after all.

All that smiling and celebrating, all that good cheer and feeling so energized—all of it goes away in an instant. My self-love evaporates before my eyes. As we ride upward together, I can't help thinking: *I can't win. The minute I get on an elevator with a gorgeous woman, I become nothing. And she's got to be around my age. Arrgh!*

11

Probably a kept woman, I reason. I begin to point out her invisible flaws in a futile attempt to make myself feel better. *No one is naturally that thin* and *healthy. I'm sure she is miserable on the inside. I mean, she must practically starve herself.* I know better than this, of course. I'm a Life Coach, for Pete's sake. These are not exactly high-minded thoughts, and don't think that's not driving me crazy. I'm lying to myself, anyway. Even if her life is a mess—even if she's the most unhappy, frustrated, and lonely woman ever to walk the face of the earth, it doesn't matter. What matters here is that I need to stop competing and comparing myself to others, and learn to appreciate myself exactly as I am.

It's then that my deepest fear begins to haunt me. . . .

Am I ever going to be good enough?

That day, I was taken aback to once again realize that no matter how much work I've done on myself, regardless of how many people I've helped to get over such self-defeating thoughts, I can still so easily be thrown off my center by comparing myself to what? . . . an image that we've all collectively labeled as "desirable" at this moment in history? It's absurd when you think about it, because what's "in" or "out" regarding beauty in our society is temporary, although far too many of us believe that the "rules" and "laws" of beauty and fashion are set in stone.

Maybe I Was Just Born in the Wrong Era

If you take ten minutes to study the history of the female body, you'll see that it's a roller-coaster of shapes and sizes, linked by several things—the amount of money people had, the clothing styles of the day, and the availability of fresh, healthy food. But there's one thing that people in all time periods had in common—the simple desire to be accepted. Everyone wants to fit in (and to fit into the latest fashions), and what other people think of as beautiful—what "the experts" and designers deem fashionable—drives the latest craze.

In the Middle Ages, a person fasted—abstaining from food completely—to be seen as spiritually enlightened. Thin was *more* than in: It was required if you wanted to be considered pious or saintly. In seventeenth-century Europe, however, large bottoms meant big pocketbooks. The rich were the only ones who could afford three hearty square meals a day, so if you didn't have the money for "good" food but you wanted to appear as though you did, you would buy the less-expensive alternative: padding with which to stuff your behind, literally.

More recently and closer to home, the height of the Twiggy era in the 1960s was on the heels of the mad obsession for wanting to look just like Marilyn Monroe. Marilyn, a curvy size 8 by today's standards (a size 12 in her day—more on that to come), was *huge* compared to Twiggy's flat-chested, 90-pound frame. During the apex of each woman's fame, however, both were desired and admired as the "ideal." And both bodies would be considered unacceptable by today's standards of ultimate health and beauty—too fat and too thin.

But just what *is* today's standard of beauty? We say we want to be fit, strong, and healthy, yet Americans spend $1 billion a year on prescription and over-the-counter weight-loss drugs. We say we want health when what we really mean, in no uncertain terms, is that we want to be thin—often at any cost. For many, smoking is a substitute for food. Others seek out laxatives and suppressants to help speed up basic bodily functions or give an added "boost."

Many experts throw blame at the entertainment and fashion industries for making otherwise healthy women body-obsessed. The media has been viewed as a factor in the dramatic increase in anorexia, bulimia, and a whole host of other body disorders, with sufficient cause.

Media campaigns spend millions and in some cases billions of dollars to appeal to our most basic human need—our desire for love. Ads show fourteen-year-old girls playing dress-up with clothes that are aimed at tempting the fashion-conscious thirty-year-old. These ads give us the impression that looking a certain way and owning a particular article of clothing or accessory will bring us happiness and, of course, the man of our dreams. They "educate" us on what styles we should wear and in what color and what fabric (styles that change from year to year), what cars we should drive, and even what our man should look like. Fashion magazines emphasize thinness as a standard for female beauty, even though their articles may try to educate us to the contrary. A picture speaks a thousand words, and we are constantly barraged by mixed messages and impossible standards.

A few facts: Most fashion models weigh 23 percent less than the average female. A twentysomething woman has about a 7 percent chance of being as slim as a catwalk model, and a 1 percent chance of being as thin as a supermodel. Yet, three-quarters of those same women say that fashion models influence their idea of the perfect body shape. With our checkbooks, we agree to accept this unrealistic body type as the dream, creating a trap for the average woman.

Here's the bottom line, and something that I can no longer ignore about myself: I can have a thousand people cheering for me and telling me that I'm beautiful and that they love me; I can feel seen, heard, and understood; I can acknowledge and be acknowledged for all my hard work, and even feel thin and sexy, but I'm *still* not enough when a skinny, gorgeous chick is standing next to me.

In that moment, it seems everyone is better, thinner, and more amazing than me. Giving up seems the only logical solution. And all my hard work, if I've been working hard, seems for naught. It feels like, once again, someone else won the beauty race. Hopelessness sets in. Pain is pain, after all. Not feeling good enough because you happen to be suddenly "trapped" inside an elevator with an über-beauty, or indulging in life-threatening substances in order to stay thin and "beautiful" are two sides of the same destructive coin.

Do I want to choose to live the rest of my life chasing beauty? No way! I no longer have the time or the inkling to wallow in the misery of comparing myself to others. And neither should you.

That said, I've seen that, even with the best of intentions, our bodies still get in our way. Over the course of the last three years, I've been changing my thoughts and habits one slow, steady step at a time. The path has been focused and purposeful, and it's been working. My best friend has told me on numerous occasions that I seem more relaxed. My sisters are amazed at my consistent effort to feel better about all parts of me. My goal never included weight loss, but it has been an unexpected and happy result. Overall, I feel more in tune with my body. It is no longer the thing that stops me, but rather it is the thing that motivates me to get outside and take a walk, to grab some veggies at work instead of a donut. In the past three years I have taken on more challenges than ever before.

What changed three years ago? Every year, like most people, I evaluate my life on January 1 and, even though I had accomplished a lot and was proud of who I had become, there was this one area that kept nagging at me: my body. I noticed that I used my body as the trump card to get me out of just about anything. And I was tired of it. I was sick of dieting and exercising. I was done hiding underneath layers of clothing. I had used my body as an excuse to stay single, stay home, and stay small. It was a new year and I was ready for a new me.

What was my intention? I remember my exact words: "I no longer want my body to stop me from living the life my soul intended." I wanted to feel happy to be alive. I wanted to be healthy — really healthy. I wanted to be an adventure girl. I wanted to be naked with a man without cringing, to dance with my nephew at his wedding and not feel too old to do a whirl, and to let myself start expressing myself through my body. I wanted it all.

I have to say I had no real idea what a "new me" meant three years ago, but I do now. I'm really learning to love myself, and people tell me it shows. Not just in the way I carry myself, but in my eyes, in my expressions, and in my energy. Not all days are good days, for sure. I still wrestle with old demons, and so will you. But life continues to get better all the time. To me, that is more valuable than anything.

Ask yourself: What is your intention? Why read a book on body image? What do you really want to gain? Learn? Lose? Tell the truth.

When you are willing to be honest with yourself, you are putting your heart before your ego. You are saying that you matter. The truth isn't always easy, but it's always the best place to start. So I have another question for you. . . .

Taking Inventory

When you look in the mirror, do you feel beautiful?
Confident?
Powerful?

Sexy?

If not, why not?

I've asked countless people what's stopping them from feeling great in their own skin, and one answer is repeated over and over again. . . .

"*My body,*" they say. Some speak the words without a second thought. Like it's a matter of fact. Others almost whisper them, fearful that they'll appear shallow, ashamed that they haven't learned to control it, change it, manage it.

"*No matter what my weight, no matter what size I wear, there is always something about my body I don't like,*" they continue, almost verbatim what I've heard a thousand times before. For some, it's a specific area that they feel ruins it for the rest of their body. It might be the size of their ankles or their unsightly upper arms or the way their back flab bulges at their bra line. When they're having a bad day, their body is to blame. A good day, on the other hand, happens in spite of their body. For others, the list of complaints is long, and their mood, hopeless. What's the point, they argue. They can't change their body; there's just too much to try to fix.

I know the feeling. If someone gave me a dark chocolate candy bar for every time I've said or thought, *Oh, if only my body were different, then I could be happy, fall in love, and make more money,* I could fill up every child's pillowcase in California on Halloween.

You've heard the stats. We all have. According to the Centers for Disease Control and Prevention, the average American woman is five foot four, weighs 163 pounds, wears a size 14, and is considered overweight by today's standards. With more than half of Americans overweight, and 1 out of every 3 of those considered obese, we're left with approximately 30 percent who are considered "normal weight."

And of those, I doubt if more than 1 percent of them are happy in their own skin.

We Americans are obsessed with our body image. We're fixated with thoughts of changing our form, wondering if it can be changed, and hoping it will change itself. Yet, we are a nation totally disassociated with our bodies and how to love them. We're in denial about how to talk to ourselves in empowering ways, how to effectively exercise and nurture ourselves, and how to deal with our stress and emotions. We think our body needs to be fixed, and we pray that the next diet or pill or magical cream or surgical procedure will be the answer.

Warning! This is *not* a weight-loss book, although weight-loss certainly may be a by-product of what I share. I am not going to give you an exercise regime or a list of vitamins to take in these pages. I will not be giving you the cure for eating disorders or the secret to what lies behind your cravings. You may receive some of those benefits naturally, as chapter by chapter you confront your body beliefs. But those are *results*—and today I want you to focus on the *process*. The process of how you've been attacking, betraying, and denying your body with the abusive decisions you make, and then the *process* of getting over yourself and getting on with your life. Sound good?

I'm going to go out on a limb here and share something that might surprise you: ***Your negative body image has little to do with your actual body!*** Study after study has proven that our body hatred isn't about the number on the scale or the ticks on the measuring tape. It is about our lack of worth, our diminished sense of self, and the lies we tell ourselves. That was definitely true for Christie.

How Did It Get to This?

Christie entered the *Starting Over* house because she thought that if she could just be beautiful, all her problems would be solved. Men would want her. The beauty industry would discover her and make her famous. Riches would be hers. She would have everything she ever imagined if she could just figure out a way to get the body of her dreams.

Christie, however, had a food addiction and a lazy mentality. She didn't want to exercise to gain her perfect body; she thought it would happen by magic. So she ate when she was lonely, drank when she was scared, and generally punished her body for not being perfect from the start. She reached her highest weight of 267 pounds and realized she wanted out of her unconscious lifestyle, but didn't know where to start. Her solution? Gastric bypass surgery, a tummy tuck, and a boob job.

When she entered the *Starting Over* house, I asked her how she had thought her body would change after surgery. Her answer: "I would have the perfect body."

But it never happened. Sure, she lost more than 120 pounds, but that wasn't enough. To Christie having the "perfect" body meant being a size 6 with ample breasts, a thin waist, and a tight butt. But after her surgery, like most miracle seekers, she never exercised, she see-sawed between eating right and eating poorly, she never gave up drinking, and she stayed in unhealthy relationships that lowered her self-esteem. Her solution? More surgery. This time around, an arm reduction.

Christie wanted to wear sleeveless blouses, but due to her rapid weight loss, she acquired loose skin on her arms. She wanted to have it cut off, and did so. But the surgeon was too eager, and her quest for beautiful, thin, sculpted biceps resulted in two uneven arms, with scars that ran from her elbows to her armpits.

Her dream of the perfect body was ruined, *"Unless,"* she thought . . .

"I'll just get a lower lift, liposuction on my thighs, and redo my arms."

During my first coaching session with Christie, she admitted that she wanted more plastic surgery, and a wave of sadness hit me. This young, beautiful girl before me had no idea what it meant to be beautiful. *If she could just look at herself in the mirror with no judgment, she would stop her senseless quest for perfection and embrace the body she already had.* But I knew getting there wouldn't be easy.

Christie wanted to be part of that small percentage of women that reaches the phantom ideal, even if it meant giving up her health to do so. It was clear to me that the solution to higher self-esteem wouldn't be more plastic surgery or radical diets. Instead, Christie needed to reevaluate why she wanted to be perfect and what her quest for perfection was really about. What was she hiding? What was she running away from? What was she, or any of us, trying to ignore? (In the chapters to come, you'll see more than a few of my reasons.)

Just like Christie, few of us have the courage to ask ourselves why we obsessively want a different body. Yes, it's natural, even healthy, to aspire to feel better and desire to be healthier, but I believe our obsessions often arise because we don't want to deal with the real reason for our unhappiness: a failed marriage, an unhappy childhood, a lost love, disappointment for how life has turned out for us, resentment at having to grow up, a job or career we don't want. Our body has the unfortunate distinction of being an easy distraction that can pull us away from the real problems in our lives.

Let's face it: self-loathing, negative thoughts, body hatred, and low body confidence can create a myriad of superficial problems that seem to take up a lot of time, leaving us little energy to heal our hearts and attend to the things that truly matter. In simplistic terms, a poor body image is a symptom of deeper issues.

Why do I feel so fat? is a question we must all answer for ourselves, sometimes on a daily basis. It is a question you'll be asking yourself and answering throughout this book as we cover many different aspects of body image. Christie has started this inquiry, and her answers reflect concerns she has had since childhood: an all-pervasive loneliness, anger at her mother for a long-term drug dependency, her own attraction to abusive boyfriends, an unfulfilling career, and so on.

As often happens with my clients, Christie tried to convince me that she had dealt with these past hurts already. She really wanted to believe that she had. But like most people, she was disconnected from her pain. Her life events had become just a bunch of stories she told herself, with little emotional connection to the actual experience. Intellectually she knew something was still wrong (her first hint was that most of her friends weren't cutting up their arms), but she never let herself feel the hurt and the emptiness that went along with those heartbreaks. That would just be too painful, too hard. Instead, Christie's so-called body "problems" conveniently occupied all her time.

Over and over I tell the women in the *Starting Over* house that the feeling you refuse to feel is the feeling that is running your life. That's why it's so essential to do this healing work.

Do you feel fat, regardless of the number on the scale? Do you hide your body, even though you know you shouldn't? Do you abuse your body with unhealthy actions? If so, why? Because you, like Christie, have a feeling you don't want to feel, an experience you want to avoid at all costs, a sense of shame about who you really are. But, as you probably know by now, it's impossible to be happy while you are hiding. Until you embrace your whole life as your own, you will never be truly free. You will never be your best, or get on with your life.

Your Exercise

Ask yourself:

How would my life change if I embraced my body just as it is, accepted my body just as it is, and loved my body just as it is? Imagine being free to express yourself fully through your body. That might mean exercising with friends in the morning, going swimming at a public pool, riding waves at the beach, dancing to music with people watching, going on a date, hugging without worrying about doing it right, and even having the best sex of your life. Go ahead. Answer the question. *How would your life change?*

Complete the following sentence:

If I embraced my body as it is, accepted my body as it is, and loved my body as it is, I could:

_____

_____

Does your answer frighten you? Mine did, and so did Christie's. That's okay. Being free *sounds* good as a passing thought, but the actual experience is scary for most of us. When Christie looked truthfully at the question above, her answer was profound. Embracing her body as is, accepting her body as is, and loving her body as is would give her the courage to face the things she had been trying to ignore. She'd be able to quit blaming her mother for abandoning her, to grieve the father who died when she was five, to give up codependent relationships, and to quit using her weight as an excuse to stay in a job that was unsatisfying.

What would that mean for her everyday life? Christie would actually have to face what lay beneath the pounds, and for her, as well as many people dealing with the issues that cause their body dissatisfaction, that seemed even harder than continuing to deny what got her here. Christie had wasted a lot of time being unhappy with herself, and that unhappiness had led to different numbing behaviors (the over-consumption of alcohol, a prescription painkiller addiction, and bulimia). But she came to see that avoiding the obvious was only a function of her fear. She came to see that denial is never a good long-term action plan.

No More, My Friend

We're all guilty of overlooking the needs of our bodies in some way, at some time. In my distant past, I used alcohol to numb my pain. Nowadays, I tend to abuse myself by not getting enough sleep, working myself into a frenzy, and comparing myself to the Victoria's Secret catalog models (yikes). I often reach for comfort foods when what I really need is rest and nutrition. But I've been changing these patterns, and so can you. First off, you need to see where it is that you abuse your body, and realize that hurting yourself is a way to validate your fears and forget your dreams.

That behavior, my friend, stops today. Hurting yourself is no longer acceptable. Through reading this book, and doing each and every exercise, you'll discover how to embrace your body, and hopefully learn to accept and eventually even love it.

Stop and reread that last sentence. I am asking you to consider embracing the body you have right *now*, accept the body you have right *now* and even, perhaps, love the body you have right *now*. If that is unacceptable to you, I dare you to read on. If that seems impossible to you, let me assure you that it is not. If you are repulsed by the thought of embracing your body, I urge you to continue. Your freedom lies within these pages.

One of the first things I did with Christie was to help her face her desire to be perfect. She's not alone. Many of us are on a quest for body perfection, while others have given it up on the surface, but still cling to the belief that if only their bodies were different, their lives would be so much better.

That desire has been running many of our lives, but everything's about to change. . . .

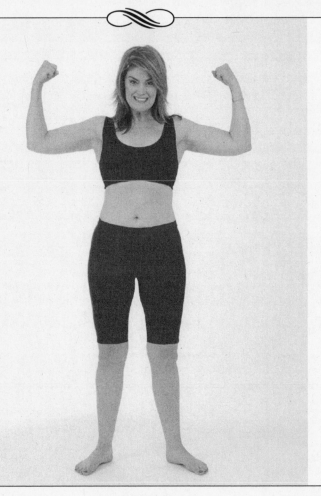

ANDY

Height: 5'10½" • Weight: 161 pounds • Age: 35

Body Motto: *I'm a big-boned girl who rarely skips dessert . . . why should I, when a better bra, great-fitting jeans, and a fabulous pair of heels can make me look ten pounds thinner?*

CHAPTER 2

What Does My Perfect Body Look Like?

There is nothing wrong with wanting to look your best. I strive to on a regular basis, and under most circumstances, my efforts pay off and I feel good about my looks. But it seems like every worry, anxiety, or fear I have ever had about my body suddenly pops up when a special event looms ahead on the horizon. Looking my "best" takes on new meaning, and the number on the scale becomes amplified in its importance. I want to look *more* than my best; I want to be slim and trim and, well, here goes that darn word again . . . p-e-r-f-e-c-t.

All of my deepest fears were brought to the forefront one recent rainy day in New York City. I was visiting for the weekend and I was on a mission: to find a dress to wear to the Emmy Awards. Allow me to set the scene. It's the first time *Starting Over* has been nominated for an Emmy and I'm obsessed with the "What ifs." *What if* Starting

Over *wins? What if I have to walk to the podium to accept my first Emmy Award? What if I trip? What if we're sitting there, cameras capturing our every breath as we're waiting to hear the outcome, and we lose? What if I look like a loser? I don't want to look like a loser! And on it goes. What if my future husband is in the audience? What if he isn't? What if I don't lose weight? What if I gain weight? What if I can't find a dress that hides my arms, covers my butt, and shows off my cleavage?*

I lay my "What ifs" at stylist Andy Paige's feet and she assures me, promises me, really, that I will look great. "Calm down, honey," she coos, as she's done before. "You're going to look beautiful. You've got my word." One of the original six women in the first *Starting Over* house in Chicago, Andy entered the house as an ex-plus-size model and failed TV style reporter, but since her graduation, she has become the CEO of her own company, Cents of Style. Today she travels the country helping women everywhere look like a million bucks without spending a fortune. She and I have become more than client and coach; we have become friends. I help her with her business dealings and she helps me with my "look." Personally, I think I'm getting the better end of the deal.

In the business of show business, sadly, much of what you show to the world is your body. My challenge, until very recently, has been to hide as much of me as I could, but Andy's been helping me expose myself by teaching me how to best maximize my assets and minimize my self-consciousness.

So with Andy's good cheer and endless expertise on all things style-related, we begin trudging through the streets of New York City with a singular goal in mind. Before nightfall, we're going to have found and purchased the most beautiful Emmy dress possible. It'll fit like a glove, be one-of-a-kind, and be more than comfortable enough to wear for the whole four-hour event without any hint of a wardrobe malfunction. We don't have much time, but the real issue worrying me at this point is that we're on a budget. Yuck. I'm not a great budgeter in the first place, but Andy's work is built around the motto that she can dress anyone beautifully for $100 or less. I'm not about to mess with her business model by spending a fortune on a dress I'll only wear once . . . but this *is* the Emmys! Definitely not the time to pinch pennies. So, without straying too far from her bargain-dressing formula, we decide that I can spend up to $500. The minute we make the agreement, I'm feeling woozy.

In order to obtain the ultimate "look" in store after store, Andy enlists the aid of a helpful salesclerk and begins describing my body in excruciating detail. "Rhonda is fleshy (my interpretation: fat) with a curvy figure (my perception: not enough waist). We need to find something that accents her cleavage (yes, she actually says that) while minimizing her tummy and covering her upper arms (I hear: because they jiggle). Yet it has to be short enough to show off her legs (hallelujah)."

I am standing still, pretending to be unaffected by this in-depth scrutinizing by Andy, the salesclerk, and any passerby patrons. What I really want to do is run to the sleepwear section, rip about 100 bathrobes off their hangers, and bury myself under a comforting pile of chenille where I can fantasize that I'm twenty years old again with a body to die for. *"Please God,"* I whisper under my breath as the woman with the pesky tape measure wraps her arms uncomfortably around my belly, *"I ask you to forgive me for hating my body back when I was thin and in shape. I promise to take better care of this one, now. I promise to honor what I've got. Just please help me find something that fits so this torture will end."*

I have complete confidence that God answers prayers. But not always exactly or as quickly as I would like, because right now, with each dress I try on, my humiliation grows. The gorgeous black one won't fit over my breasts. Well, that's not totally accurate. I've got it on, finally, but my girls are sticking out in bumpy lumps. The silky blue one has fabric that won't quite stretch far enough around my midsection. "No. No. No," Andy says, as if it's become her new mantra. A little red number looks like it might be the one, but then I turn around. My behind looks twice its size. Again, Andy pleadingly outlines my glaringly obvious limitations to the clerk, "Don't you have *anything*?" This time it's the clerk's turn to say no.

As night falls, we've ransacked ten stores and we're reaching the end of our time together, not to mention that I'm at the end of my rope. You'd think finding a dress for the Emmys would be a dream come true. You'd think a slew of designers would pounce, wanting, begging, to dress me. The truth is I'm on a daytime reality show, walking around in a size 8 body. (Samples, which are given out freely, are usually in a size 6 and mostly offered first to the stars of nighttime TV.) The irony is that I'm "too big" physically, yet "too small" of a name (meaning that I'm not yet high-wattage enough) for the designers to take notice.

I try to keep a positive attitude in the midst of my growing anxiety. The "What ifs" begin their second assault. *What if we go to every store in Manhattan and there's nothing? What if I have to wear my old "at least it fits" black dress from ten years ago that I bought when I officiated at a friend's wedding? (It's faded and has a hole under the left arm.) What if I have to have a dress made? Who will do it? What fabric would I use?* Andy sees my eyes glaze over. "We're going to Bergdorf Goodman," she announces, jolting me back to the present.

Bergdorf Goodman is *the* store in New York City for fancy

dresses—dresses that cost an arm and a leg, by the way. But I'm desperate, and realizing that looking good, really good, doesn't come cheap. We both know my budget's going to be blown, but this is quite possibly a once-in-a-lifetime event, and the photos will follow me for the rest of my life. Even Andy admits that it's worth the investment. We arrive, and the melodic sounds of the overhead speakers instantly calm my nerves. It feels good in here. Peaceful. Abundant. They've *got* to have what we're looking for.

The couture saleswoman starts off by showing us Prada, Chanel, and other designers whose names I can't pronounce, let alone have even heard of. Andy grabs an armload of possibilities and we make our way to what I'm hoping will be the final changing room of the day. It looks like the Rolls Royce of dressing rooms, complete with two three-way mirrors, until I notice the strange lighting that seems to accentuate my every bulge. As I strip down to my underwear, all I see is rolls and ripples and chunks. It's like they've got magnifiers right in the glass! I'm no longer feeling so peaceful and wonder why they even bothered to pump in the soothing tunes. Why not just screech a little heavy metal over the loudspeakers? Shopping for an Emmy dress makes bathing suit shopping—once my least favorite pastime—seem like child's play.

And then it happens: Magic. I slip on a deep-blue crepe dress with a plunging neckline and bell skirt and I look amazing. Like I've lost twenty pounds! Andy squeals. This is it. I breathe a sigh of relief and check myself up and down, backward and forward, front to back. Sure enough, there's no mistaking it. My body looks hot! The color brings out my eyes. My skin is glowing. My arms even look thin. I glance at the price tag. $10,000! Holy cow. I look at Andy. She looks at the price tag. We scream. This was not part of the plan!

My mind is whirling. How can a smart, educated, even "successful" woman who has been actively working on her body image consciously fall prey to such temptation? I know better—just barely—than to write out a check like this. And I know that I can't compare my body to the body of the actors who walk down the red carpet. They wear $10,000 dresses because they get them for *free*; because their careers are built around being sexy, because they are paid millions of dollars a film. Who am I kidding?

The fact that I even contemplated pulling out a credit card for that $10,000 dress for a four-hour event confirms how I felt in that moment: Fat. Ugly. Desperate. Anything but perfect.

An Ugly Secret

Unless you're in fashion, and even if you are, you may not know that until the 1950s, every garment we wore was hand-sewn. Our mothers or grandmothers purchased a pattern or made one themselves, took our measurements, picked the fabric, and sewed the pieces together. We might have tried on that garment two or three times before it was cleared to be worn. Clothes were made to fit our individual bodies perfectly and, therefore, they FIT. This is no longer the case. With mass production, ready-to-wear garments, and the invention of the "fit model," a system has been put in place that has perhaps caused more disappointment for women than our search for Mr. Right.

Fit models are a peculiar bunch. To the fashion industry, they are considered the models of perfection. They are women, just like you and me, except that they have a specific body type that will, as long as they're modeling for that clothing line, forever be the form those clothes will take. Their shape, be it small-breasted or narrow-hipped, will become the basis for the sizing of that clothing manufacturer's garments. Fit models are either size 8 or size 12, depending on the clothing line. If the line goes up to size 14 and down to size 2, a size 8 fit model is smack-dab in the middle. (A size 12 fit model is used when a clothing line is focused on satisfying the full figure. Catalogs aimed at larger ladies will only use up to size 14 models to sell their clothing because studies have shown that women will only buy clothes if the model is no bigger than size 14.) When Andy was a perfect size 12, she was a fit model for two reasons: small breasts and "boy hips." Manufacturers loved her body: With few body curves to deal with, they get away with using less fabric, and consequently fewer man-hours because in making fewer darts, they lower their costs. That means that in order for clothes by that manufacturer to fit you or me like a glove right off the rack, we must have small breasts and boy hips. I don't know about you, but I have neither.

The less expensive and more mass-produced a garment, the fewer tucks and pleats and darts it will have. With my curvy body, I'm just plain out of luck. I think of all the years I thought I was fat when I tried on clothes at my local department store. I had no idea that without their cookie-cutter body type, I didn't have a chance. That size 8 fit model would be the basis for sizes 2, 4, 6, 10, 12, and 14 (by merely adding or subtracting two inches between sizes). I wouldn't have found a fit no matter what size I became, because my natural body type would not fit into their idea of perfection.

How can any woman win the battle of the unfit bathing suit, the ridiculously snug pants bottom, or the baggy bodice? I understand the clothing manufacturers are just trying to make a buck, but this is insanity! How are we ever supposed to look our best?

Girdles Galore

Back in New York, I've decided not to mortgage my home to buy "the perfect dress" . . . but I still need something to wear for the biggest night of my life. Andy has the solution, and I get excited just looking at her mischievous grin. "Time to get a corset," she says. On our way to yet another store's lingerie section, she explains that the reason the $10,000 dress sucks me in and flattens my tummy, making me feel like a million bucks, is because its foundation is an inner corset. We are going to find the right "foundation garments" (my interpretation: girdles) to recreate what we were experiencing with the I-wish-I-could-afford-you expensive dress. I sheepishly follow her to Macy's department store, hoping I'll find the answer to my "problem."

Making our way through the racks of tummy slimmers and bust enhancers, Andy pulls out a one-piece body suit, a corset-type bustier, and a knee-to-bust Miracle Slimmer Suit. And then she tells me to put on all three . . . at the same time! First, I tug up the one-piece body suit using my hand to squish in my waist and pull up my breasts. Next, Andy puts the corset bustier around my waist and starts tightening. I can barely breathe, but I don't say a word— I just want to buy a dress. Finally, I step into the girdle of all girdles: the Miracle Slimmer Suit. I mention to her that all these garments must add inches to my frame, so won't this actually make me look bigger? She scoffs and grabs the back of the girdle and hikes it up my butt. "There," she exclaims, "that looks better."

I see my image staring back at me in the full-length mirror. Has it come to this? Am I that fat that I have to wear three, count them, *three* girdles in order for a dress to fit? She hands me a bright green satin dress that I slip over my head and voilà, it's perfect. I see that being my best isn't my best at all, but a manufactured version of it. I feel simultaneously defeated and elated. I have a dress, one that is well below the original $500 ceiling I set for myself. But I have to admit that when all was said and done, my body image was in the toilet.

My search for my Emmy dress brought up feelings that I had worked hard at healing. I was thrown for a loop by how vulnerable and insecure I still was. Hadn't I given up reading the message boards? Hadn't I been working out faithfully for two years? Hadn't I been taking vitamins to fortify my body? Hadn't I emptied my refrigerator of Betty Crocker vanilla whipped frosting, Ben & Jerry's Phish Food ice cream, and frozen pizzas? Hadn't I been getting educated and, more importantly, helping other women get over their own body issues?

The answer was yes. I had been doing better on a day-to-day basis, but this "big" event was outside my comfort zone. I always tell the women of the *Starting Over* house that new situations will bring up old behaviors and old addictions, so be attentive when crisis hits. While the Emmys weren't a crisis situation, I was still more nervous than I was used to. And thinking negatively about my body has always had an addictive quality to it. Once I start, I have a hard time stopping.

Other big events can take on the feeling of a crisis situation. They usually involve being seen by loads of people, stepping into a situation where you have less control than normal, and can include people from your past who often seemed to judge you. A high school reunion, a family get-together, an old flame's wedding, or even a much-needed vacation can bring up feelings of inadequacy and betrayal. I felt inadequate because no matter how much I had been working out or eating right, in the mirror at Macy's that day it didn't seem to matter. I felt betrayed by a body that wouldn't respond in the way I thought it should.

Just like yours, my quest for perfection came with a price tag. It cost me more than the sum total of three girdles, one dress, one pair of shoes, and a bevy of accessories. It cost me my self-esteem. With little self-esteem, who could blame me for skipping an event or two? Isn't that what you and I say to ourselves? Some version of, *"I'm not up for it,"* or *"Not tonight; I don't feel good,"* or, *"I'm too tired."*

What has your quest for perfection cost you? Take a minute. Don't rush to answer, because I want you to be truthful. What has your desire to be different, better, or more than yourself cost you in terms of your health? Relationships? Career? Confidence? How have you held yourself back and closed the doors to waiting opportunities?

In the past, because of my desire to be so much better than I was, I had given up on dating, convinced that the men I'd want wouldn't want me looking like I did. In my career, I had also given up on opportunities, thinking I wasn't ready because my body wasn't. Feeling powerful and empowered? Oh, my body—or rather my thoughts about my body—cost me that as well. These losses are common to many of us, a truth which has become clear to me since coaching others, but specifically through working in the *Starting Over* house.

Outlining Your Perfect Body

A woman named Summer moved into the *Starting Over* house in the second season, and I immediately identified with her. She, too, had lost a lot because of her beliefs and negative habits. According to her, she had lost herself. Summer also wanted to be perfect (a repeating theme here), and that desire had nearly paralyzed her motivation. In order to get close to the perfection she sought, Summer knew it was finally time to deal with her ups and downs concerning her obesity. She loved her grandmother and confessed that her grandmother's obesity made her realize that if she didn't do something fast, she could end up just like her—ill and in the hospital. But, more importantly, Summer worried about dying alone. She was afraid of never getting married or having a family. Wanting to experience romance, intimacy, and eventually motherhood, she believed that losing her excess weight was a necessary component toward realizing those goals.

But wanting something and attaining it are very different. As her Life Coach in the house, I knew that Summer did her best to compensate for her negative body image by working harder than anyone else. Her fragile self-esteem had survived because she had successfully combined her strong work ethic with a job she loved. She was good at something and was acknowledged for it. Summer was also wise enough to realize that once she reached her ideal goal weight, she'd have a new set of hurdles to jump. In some respects, living her life as the chubby girl was comfortable, and she knew that being thin would present higher stakes and a whole new set of challenges.

For one of Summer's first exercises in the *Starting Over* house, I asked her to answer the following question: *If you could have the perfect body, what would it look like?* With a black Magic Marker in hand, Summer drew her dream body: an hourglass figure, labeled with words like *empowered, beautiful,* and *thin.* It was svelte and sexy, with measurements that could rival any model's.

Summer's Perfect Body:

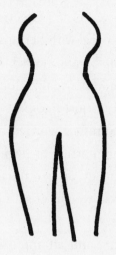

empowered

beautiful

thin

Summer's ideal body is close to my ideal, except I have a few additional adjectives like *toned, fit, healthy,* and *loved.*

Your Exercise

I ask you the same question. ***If you could have the perfect body, what would it look like?*** Be as specific as possible with your answer. I urge you to be more than your usual honest. It's time to be super honest. Don't draw the body you think you can have. Draw the body you WANT to have—your perfect body. Go ahead and draw it below, and label it with the feelings you believe you would experience if you had that body today.

My Perfect Body Looks Like . . .

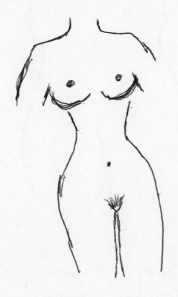

Sexy
Confident
healthy
energetic
strong)

Good job!

As soon as I knew exactly how Summer *wanted* to feel about herself, it was time to find out how she actually felt in that moment. I asked Summer to draw her body as it was. What did she imagine it looked like to the outside world? As I expected, she drew a chunky, androgynous-looking body, with few curves. She labeled it with words like *genderless, depressed,* and *sad.* That's how Summer really saw herself. At her current weight, she felt "sexless," which told me that she felt unwanted. Unlovable. Very much alone.

Summer's Body Now:

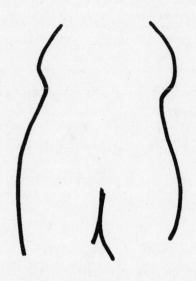

genderless   sexless

depressed   unlovable

sad   alone

After completing her second drawing, I knew that we had uncovered Summer's level of body distortion—where the reality of her body differed from her perceptions. Summer thought her body was disgusting, but that wasn't true. Yes, she was overweight for her height and body frame, and yes, she was walking a thin line between healthy and unhealthy, but that didn't take away from the fact that she was beautiful. Her eyes sparkled, her smile was contagious, and she was friendly, open, and kind. She carried her weight well, and in fact, if I didn't know better I would have thought that

Summer loved her body. She wore sleeveless shirts and colorful out-fits that advertised a woman who was anything but plagued by self-loathing. She walked tall, looked people in the eyes, and seemed to have a strong sense of self. But inside she was condemning herself, and it didn't matter what I saw or what I said. (It never matters what others say when you don't choose to believe in yourself.) I could compliment Summer until the cows came home, and I did, but un-til she wanted to believe me, chose to believe me, and did believe me, my praises fell on deaf ears. I was hoping that through our work together, Summer would soon be able to see her inner and *outer* beauty.

I know Summer's just like millions of you out there now—part of the beautiful, talented, loving women who are so busy seeing their negatives that they don't understand how incredibly valuable and beautiful they are—to their children, their friends, their husbands, parents, coworkers, bosses, and clients. If we're honest with our-selves, we'll admit that there are many times we feel genderless, hopeless, or even lifeless—no matter how many people love us and want us.

Your Exercise

How do you perceive your body as it is right now? Go ahead and draw the body you think the world sees. Be honest. This is no time to lie, exaggerate, or fudge (*and I don't mean the yummy kind*). Do it if you truly want to get over your body and on with your life.

Your Body Now:

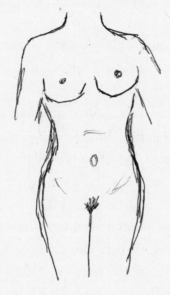

real
Chubby
Tired
less

How does it feel to draw your body? Was it easy or hard, or did you skip the drawing altogether, convinced that this silly exercise couldn't really make a difference? Drawing your body takes courage. It takes a willingness to face one of your greatest fears. This exercise isn't for the faint of heart; it's for the woman who wants to be fearless.

What words did you use to describe yourself? Were you willing to be vulnerable in your description of how you really feel about your body?

I understand that you may have days where you are grateful for your body, and maybe even love it. Congratulations. But I want to know about all of your days. The good, the bad, and the indifferent.

So again, look at the picture that you drew of your body. Be sure to write down everything you feel about it, and be sure to attach words to the drawing. The more truthful you are, the more the work we do together will make a difference.

Size Really Doesn't Matter

Unrealistic expectations and body denial are two ways we keep ourselves stuck in body hatred. If we believe we have to have the perfect body to be happy, our expectations will never be met and our good intentions will evaporate with our self-esteem. If you had the perfect body, which, remember, changes like the wind, I absolutely know that you'd find something else to be unsatisfied with. Thinking that happiness resides in a size 2 or a size 6 or a size 12 is why "vanity sizing" thrives. Vanity sizing is when ready-to-wear manufacturers shift size 12 to size 10, and so on. You have the illusion, based on the size you purchase, of being smaller than you are, but your body hasn't changed at all. "Designer delusion" is the same thing, but reserved for the lines of clothing that are pricier. The higher the price of your garment, the more you will be assured that their guarantee is firmly in place: You'll think you are thinner without lifting a weight. This is what causes "designer loyalty" and "shopping without stopping"— wearing a size 2 when you actually wear a size 6 feels so good. We become seduced with the promise that in *their* line of clothing we will be our dream size. We *will* be perfect.

Unless you are willing to work for a healthier body, all the denying and expectations in the world won't change how you feel about you. Most of us treat the "temple of our soul" like an object rather than a living, breathing entity. Think about it: We wouldn't stuff our Scottish terrier into a doghouse that's too small, and we

43

wouldn't put our cat in a collar that's two sizes too big. But we stuff ourselves into clothing that is restrictive, imagining that if it "fits," we will look good. Or we get lost, drowning in clothes that are larger than our frame, all because we want to hide our body underneath layers of fabric, hoping no one is looking. We don't pay attention to the fit of our clothes because if we did, we'd have to face the reality of our shape. And for many of us, denial is a better place to be.

When Andy Paige and I find ourselves in the same town, she helps me shop for the wardrobe I wear on *Starting Over*. During our last shopping trip, I purchased a size 12 pair of pants, a size 6 blouse, a size 8 dress, and a size 0 sports jacket. Before I learned about designer delusion and vanity sizing, I would never have tried on the size 0 jacket or the size 6 blouse. I would have assumed they would be too small. What Andy taught me is that size truly doesn't matter. The only thing that matters is fit, and since I now know a portion of all clothing is mis-sized due to manufacturing error, I have more courage to grab any size on the rack. Because when a garment fits, it feels perfect on the body you have, not the body you are secretly waiting for.

When shopping for the Emmy dress, and in my first trips to find a wardrobe for the show, not being able to just grab something off the rack triggered my feelings of failure. Even though I had recently lost ten pounds, I felt fat all over again. It didn't seem fair. Even though I was armed with the history of the fit model and the knowledge of how the clothing industry doesn't sew for my body type, logic went out the window. I felt like a victim and I didn't care about the reasons why. I just wanted something, anything, to fit. Because if it fits, I fit in, somehow. In trying on dresses that didn't fit, I was reminded of how I never really felt like I fit in.

There it is. In a chunky, little nutshell. One of the feelings I don't want to feel: That I don't belong. Belonging is my core need, something we all silently search for. When I don't belong, I feel powerless, helpless, and out of control. These are the feelings I felt growing up. Feelings I have learned to master over the years, allowing everything to be all right with my world. And, when I get enough sleep and eat right, I am mostly stress-free. But the minute I work too much, or lose an hour of sleep, or take on more than I can handle, my feelings quickly shift and become harder to hide.

We all want to belong because we all want to feel loved.

At the conclusion of our first coaching session, I told Summer what I am about to tell you: Your desire to be perfect is stopping you from experiencing the very love you so desperately want to feel. Having a perfect body does not guarantee love, but a healthy body image does. So it's up to you: Chase the dream of perfection or experience self-love.

Your willingness to embrace your humanity will set you free from the media-obsessed version of who you think you are supposed to be. Just like you, I have my thin days, my fat days, and my oh-my-gosh-shut-the-blinds days. If I watch myself on the television, I have to take a few deep breaths or it definitely cuts into my self-esteem. But if I work out, eat right, and get good sleep, I automatically feel better about my life, including the shape of my body. The type of day I am having does *not* have to be decided by the size of my body. The question comes down to: Am I willing to embrace the body I have and experience self-love, or will I wait until everything is perfect and hope I feel loved by everyone (including myself)?

Helping you answer that question is the purpose of this book. I don't want the size or the label on the back of my favorite pair of pants to hold any importance. What I want to matter is love. Love of self. Love of others. Love of life. But for most people, like Summer, too much is standing in the way, namely an unrealistic idea of perfection. It doesn't count if we lie to ourselves, saying that we've given up the dream, because if we truly had, our body would be our friend, our companion, our ally.

In the end, Summer chose love. She discovered that when a person's body quits being his or her excuse, so many more options and possibilities open up. That can be overwhelming and intimidating, but also very freeing. I understand the fear of change all too well. It's the reason many people fail when they attempt to embrace their body. Feeling good about yourself is not always welcomed, especially if you have used your negative body image as the excuse for all your problems. Just know that the path that lies before you will be fraught with inspiration, motivation, and some tears. You will never be the same.

Oh, did I mention that we won the Emmy that night? And yes, my three girdles and I held up beautifully. As I stood holding my gleaming statue, I could hardly believe how blessed I was—an insecure girl from the Midwest being honored for changing people's lives. If my dreams can come true, yours can, too! Of course, you have to believe . . .

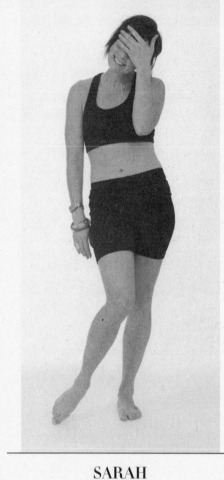
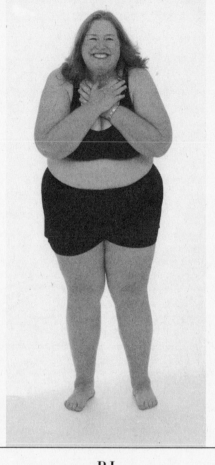

SARAH
Height: 5'5"
Weight: 125 pounds
Age: 31

BJ
Height: 5'5"
Weight: 300 pounds
Age: 55

Same Hidden Belief: *I'm never going to look like I did in my twenties, so why care now? I'm always going to look bad no matter what, so what's the use?*

CHAPTER 3

What Are My Hidden Beliefs About My Body?

I have yet to work with a woman who doesn't have a body image problem. Not a single one. People have come to me for coaching, both privately and in the *Starting Over* house, for specific help on every conceivable issue—infidelity, unresolved grief, lost love, unrequited love, broken families, stalled careers, dating dilemmas—anything you can imagine. But one thing I've learned to expect from *everyone*, male or female, young or old, is that they will have major self-confidence issues surrounding their bodies. And those insecurities will influence how they move through the world.

What do I mean by body image? It's simple, really. Body image is the perception you hold about your body. It's how you see yourself, and what you believe to be true about your body. For most of us, our body image will have little semblance to reality. What we

49

think our body looks like to the rest of the world is often very different from what others actually see and believe. We see ugly age spots, for example, when others see freckles. We see acne, when others see a few small zits. We see gross fat, when others see a little weight gain. We see hideous obesity, when others see heaviness. When others want us to come to their toga party, we stay home for fear of embarrassing ourselves. We retreat (or contort or distort) when others extend themselves because, for some reason, we just don't dare.

Sarah and BJ are perfect examples of body distortion. As you can see from their photos at the beginning of this chapter, these two women have very different body types. Sarah, lean and fit, stands five feet five inches and weighs 125 pounds. BJ, a large, robust woman, weighs in at 300 pounds and is only slightly taller than Sarah. You would think that they'd feel very differently about their bodies, but surprisingly, they are so close in their thinking processes that it's hard to tell them apart when hearing them speak about their situations.

Both women detest their bodies. Sarah can't stand looking at herself in the mirror and has convinced herself that when people see her out and about, they're secretly disgusted that she even has the courage to leave the house. BJ also just wants to hide, which may seem more relatable, considering her size and the fact that people do stare at her, children point and laugh, and men look away.

In their own way, both of these women has allowed her body to stand in the way of their happiness. Sarah tries to change her image by working out religiously, but in the end, hours on the treadmill and lifting heavy weights haven't changed how she feels. In the past year, BJ has worked diligently on facing her fears. She has spoken up in groups, been fitted by a bra specialist, and has volunteered to have the photo taken you see today. By facing her issues and expressing them out loud, BJ feels healthier, stronger, and more beautiful for it. Sarah, on the other hand, is still battling with the image she wants for herself—still hoping for some elusive state of perfection that's all in her head. If she's unable to shift her thoughts, in a year's time, BJ may be the healthier and happier of the two women.

Just like Sarah and BJ, body image distortion gives you permission to beat yourself up and put yourself down. In reality, most folks imagine that they're heavier than they really are. You'd think that would be good news . . . that we'd all realize the error of our ways and run to the scales to pat ourselves on the back for the actual number reflected there. The reason we don't, though, is because that's not really the issue. At my thinnest, I still had a very poor body image. I would call myself names in the mirror. I would walk away in disgust when shopping for a bathing suit. I would avoid getting close to anyone, unless I was absolutely sure they loved me. (Can you imagine how much I would test and torture my partner to be assured that he really cared?) Now, as I tip the scales twenty-pounds heavier, my body image has actually improved. Go figure. What has changed?

Me.

On most days, I no longer curse my body if my jeans feel tight. I don't wait for a skinny day to go out with friends. I no longer use my body as an excuse to say no. It was a long time coming, but I've been doing something I didn't think I could do. I've started to become friends with my body. And I want the same for you.

Clearly, my shift is not because I've acquired the perfect body. I did not have plastic surgery to lift my breasts, or shell out the big dollars to have some doctor liposuction my thighs. In fact, my breasts have lost some of their buoyancy, and until only very recently, my weight didn't budge, regardless of my increasingly healthy habits.

Having a healthy body image isn't about having the *perfect* body. It's about getting over it and getting on with life.

Is It Time to Change?

Bethany woke up one day at age seventeen with total amnesia. She had no idea who she was, where she was, or what she was supposed to do about it. Her memories were gone, and even her parents and best friends had become strangers. After four years of walking around in a fog, she entered the *Starting Over* house hoping to find herself for the first time. Bethany had always felt fat, and was afraid of experiencing even trace elements of chemistry with boys. She threw herself into her singing, church, and flag team, trying not to dwell on the fact that she had never been kissed.

In working together, it soon became apparent that memory or no memory, Bethany hated her body. In her mind, it had betrayed her by being "big boned" and taller than many of the boys her age. Since getting ill, it had *really* betrayed her; the large doses of medications she was on had only added weight to her already large frame. Her recuperation time was slow and painful. We had our work cut out for us.

I knew the feeling, having felt similar shame. I finally got tired of the excuses, as did Bethany. It's a process. But let's remember that you aren't going to change until the fear and pain that comes with hiding your body is greater than the fear and pain of exposing it (with all your flaws and limitations). I'm guessing that you're at the point where you know it's time to change. Maybe you're mostly happy with your body, but you eat too many high-fat and sugary foods to give you that powerful, energized feeling that comes from being healthy and strong. Maybe you can't get through the day without four cups of coffee, and you desire the natural high that exercise brings, but haven't yet been able to create the structure to support healthy habits. Or maybe you've been undressing with the lights out for fifteen years and you finally know that nothing's going to change unless you do.

If you're really honest with yourself, you're aware that it's not just your weight that's holding you back. You see overweight people doing the things you repeatedly deny yourself. There's your chunky neighbor who wears short shorts in her side yard when she's gardening or barbecuing out back with her husband, kids, and friends. You wonder how she does it. While you're sweltering in your sweats in the Indian summer temperatures, she's giving herself the chance to be free. Then there's the woman you watched recently at the beach, sunbathing for hours with her heaviness on display for everyone to view. You never even took your dress off and she, who was a good three times your size, swam with her family and laughed and played while you felt sorry for yourself.

Do those two women love their bodies? Maybe. Maybe not. Chances are, they'd be the first ones to tell you what they don't like about their legs, their upper arms, or their jelly-roll stomachs. But, they've also stopped allowing the dislike of their individual body parts to stop them from experiencing life (at least in some situations). What I want you to get more than anything else from this book is that there's a way to treat yourself lovingly, no matter where you are in your process, no matter what the scale or the mirror shows, no matter what somebody else has to say about you.

It All Starts in the Mind

I'm guessing that you want to stop hurting yourself. You, like me, like Bethany, want to stop making excuses. You want to start feeling alive and free and healthy and, yes, even sexy. Something has happened to scare you, to capture your attention. Maybe it was when you found yourself shaking your head to another dream vacation because of your refusal to wear a bathing suit in public. You saw the look of exasperation on your husband's face, and you felt his pain at your lack of involvement. Or maybe your little girl has been begging you every Sunday to join her on the jungle gym, but you tell yourself it won't hold your weight—and besides, you get exhausted just walking to the park. Perhaps leaving your house for the farmer's market has become too much of a hassle and take-out has become your favorite food group.

Women in the *Starting Over* house have stalled their relationships, sabotaging or stopping them altogether because of negative body images. By the same token, I've seen them work hard to rewire their thinking processes and within a few months begin walking, dancing, working out, eating better, wearing more form-fitting clothes, flirting, dating—and honestly seeing themselves as desirable. Their growth has encouraged my growth, and in teaching what I've so needed to learn, I've also been reaping the rewards of healthier actions. That's why I know these ideas, exercises, and intentions will also work for you.

Saying Good-bye to Magical Thinking

Whether you like it or not, your body is yours for life. Isn't it? I mean, come on—can you really hope to trade it in for a newer model? It's a tough thing to admit—that you've been waiting for the showroom edition. Waiting for the valet to deliver it to your door. I used to hope that someday I was going to get the latest, state-of-the-art Rhonda Britten, a more svelte, toned, and overall exemplary version of the me I was given. If I just wished hard enough, prayed long enough, and complained loud enough—something would have to give. Like people who grow up believing that money grows on trees, I believed that my perfect body was just around the next corner. Surely science would catch up and make trading in the old for the new unbelievably safe, and affordable too. But eventually reality sunk in. Twenty years of bad habits weren't going to be cleared up in a day, not by science, magic, a new boyfriend, or size 0 aliens from another galaxy. I would have to get real because no matter how many imperfections I pointed out, beat myself up about, or blamed on my "faulty" genes, nothing was leading me toward self-acceptance. None of my thinking, speaking, or emoting would cause one ounce of change on my body until I committed to *do* something.

My first step was to stop living in a dream world and start seeing reality. We began the process in the previous chapter when I asked you to draw your body as it is. Now is the time to uncover the beliefs that have been holding you back. It's time to get really real.

Doing Everything All The Time

Take a look at the latest list of articles I found in a five-minute search in the more popular women's magazines:

Ten Days to a New Body
Ditch Your Diet Rules and Lose Weight
Whittle Your Middle into Bikini Shape
Gadgets that Peel Off Pounds
Your Secret Diet Weapon

*Stop Stress, Lose Weight, Love Your Life: See How Everyone Is
    Doing It!*
*Walk Off Extra Pounds: 5 Plans That'll Change Your Body
    Pronto*
6 Insider Sculpting Secrets for Sexy Abs, Butt, and Thighs

These catchy headlines seduce us with the promise of perfection, and like bees to honey, we buy into the dream because we want to believe it can happen for us. We can have the body we always wanted if we just followed the easy, step-by-step formula all these magazines have been kind enough to lay out.

I'm not knocking magazines that are trying to inform us of our body possibilities, but because we don't know any better and believe we should be able to control our bodies into submission, we end up the losers. And not the losers of pounds that we want to be. Instead, we lose portions of our self-confidence and find further reasons to blame ourselves for our glaring imperfections.

Somewhere inside of me, I had developed the belief that if I just had more self-discipline, more self-control, and more motivation, anything was possible, even, dare I say, a model-perfect body.

Here's what I was hoping (and trying) to accomplish in order to get that body:

- Exercising five days a week, making sure to get in equal parts strength training, cardiovascular workouts, and a stretching regime.
- Eating only healthy foods, never again letting sugar, salt, caffeine, or white starch touch my lips. Taking my vitamins

three times a day and getting a full eight hours of sleep, no
matter what kind of deadlines I was under.

- Drinking eight to ten glasses of water every day, without
  ever missing a day.
- Somehow having a totally positive frame of mind, where I
  would never, ever allow even the slightest negative thoughts
  about myself to enter. This would be done by reading self-
  help books in great numbers, meditating every day, taking
  long, rejuvenating walks in nature, and getting plenty of
  sun (wearing sunscreen, of course).
- Staying clear of all stress. No more negative people or
  saying yes to too many responsibilities. My boundaries
  would stay intact without exception and my time would be
  my own.

If I did all that, I was convinced I could obtain everything I
wanted and more. If I didn't, I thought I didn't deserve anything
at all, so why bother trying? If I couldn't be perfect, I was convinced I was just wasting my time.

Bethany had her own perfection plan. Some of her more strin-
gent rules included:

- Starvation: If she did break down and eat, the plainest, most
  boring vegetables and fruits were her only option. Anything
  that could be seen as desirable was off limits.
- Drinking eight to ten glasses of water every day, without
  ever missing a day.
- Smiling at all times, no matter what, so that no one knew
  how she was really feeling.

● Being perfect every day, all day. Failure was not an
  option.

Bethany believed that if she reached for a cookie, it only proved
how ridiculous her quest for perfection was. She might as well give
up, and in that moment, cakes, cookies, and potato chips were plen-
tiful. It was all or nothing.

Your Exercise

What about you? What do you think you have to do to obtain the
body you desire? Do you have to cut out sugars? Eat perfectly for
the rest of your life? What about exercise? Go ahead and list any expectations you hold about yourself. What must you do to step into
the body of your dreams? Delve as deeply as you can, and answer
the following question:

In order for me to have the best body possible, I'd have to . . .
work out 5 days a week, get enough sleep,
eat mostly healthy, Drink plenty of water,
limit - sweets, alcohol, fat, and overall
calories,

Now that you have looked at and admitted to the expectations
you have for yourself, do you still believe that your perfect body is
obtainable, regardless of your efforts (i.e. magical thinking)? Or do
you believe, like I do, that somewhere you missed the perfect-body
gene and no matter what you do, failure will be your ultimate result?

Maybe it's both of the above, and some of everything else in between. You want to believe that your hard work matters, but we've
all been there before. There are outrageous statistics that say that
90 percent of dieters regain the weight they lose. The message we

receive is that if you don't stick to your diet perfectly, you will regain the weight, and usually add on some as well. No wonder we feel defeated before we ever start.

I, too, believed I had to be at 100 percent of my best—in habits, thoughts, and looks—all the time. Then, and only then, could I accept my body because then, and only then, was I doing all that I could and therefore, deserving of the perfect body.

Earth to Rhonda . . . Wake up, Rhonda. . . . While the above scenario would be nice and in the ballpark of things you want to shoot for (overall, as in having healthy habits, thoughts, and looks), you're setting yourself up for failure if these are your expectations about what should be happening for you every day, all day.

It's essential that you look at what beliefs are running your life. Bethany believed that her body was ugly because in her mind, her weight hung around her middle like an unsightly spare tire. She had big wide calves and scars on her belly too. And because she had these "flaws," she was damaged, unfixable, and unlovable. Bethany didn't believe she was worth kissing because no boy would want her with "that" body. At twenty-one, Bethany had yet to kiss a boy.

Your Exercise

Do you believe your body is capable of achieving good health? Or do you believe you have to secretly choose between being healthy and being skinny? Are you convinced that you're stuck with your faulty genes, so there's not much you can do to change your body? Or, do you, like me, believe that you have to be perfect or it doesn't count?

Go ahead. Answer the following questions to help you come clean with your beliefs.

1. What negative thoughts (perceptions) do you have about your body? List at least five. Don't rationalize—meaning that, even if this thought's not true for you all the time, if it comes up, and you think it or feel it, write it down. Somewhere inside of you it *feels* true.

Example: One of my negative thoughts is that no one will want to be in a relationship with me with the body I have.

1. I feel invisable
2. my belly is too big
3. my stretch marks + my belly button are ugly.
4. my hair is never right.
5. my face is starting to look old + I still have zits.

2. Now that you've written down five negative thoughts, I want you to go back to each one and write down how that thought (perception) makes you feel. Attach a feeling to each previous answer.

Example: When I believe no one wants me the way I am, I feel sad, angry, and lonely.

1. invisability makes me feel sad, lonely, + unimportant
2. my big belly makes me feel frustrated + inferior
3. stretch marks arn't so bad
4. I'm always thinking if I could only fix my hair I'd look good.
5. I don't waht to look real young but I sure don't want to be old!

3. Now that you've identified some negative thoughts and their corresponding negative feelings, I want you to ask yourself what you do when you have those feelings. For each feeling, determine the action or non-action that corresponds with that feeling.

Examples: When I am sad, I eat chocolate. When I am angry, I get impatient and short with people. When I am lonely, I watch old movies and resort to eating comfort foods like cinnamon toast, pizza, and ice cream.

1. When Im invisable - I avoid people and get sadder and think Im not good enough
2. When Im frustrated about my belly I wear baggy clothes and mostly stay home.
3.
4. I keep changing my hair color, style, cut and Its sad
5.

Taking Action

There's a funny thing about actions. Actions are our response to our _feelings, not our thoughts._ Our feelings, hidden or obvious, run our lives. Those feelings come from beliefs we have about ourselves, the life we're living, and our bodies. Becoming aware of the chain reaction our beliefs have on our actions starts breaking the hold they have on the choices we make. In other words, you've got to get a hold of your feelings!

In the past, when I believed any man worth having wouldn't give me the time of day unless I had the "body beautiful," I kept intimacy at bay. That belief caused feelings of low self-worth, sadness, and anger. And those feelings gave me permission to blame my loneliness on my weight while at the same time downing a carton of Oreo cookie ice cream. Once I realized that ice cream wasn't my problem, but rather a symptom of a deeper problem, I had to interrupt the pattern. I had to do something different. I had to take a step.

Committing to a life of good health doesn't happen overnight. You must face the beliefs that have been holding you back. And you must agree to suspend those beliefs for the duration of our time together. You must be willing to accept your body as is (or at least commit to doing so), and be willing to see your body in a new light. Do you think you can do that for a few weeks or months to start? Are you willing to move toward loving the body you have and allowing others to love you?

I know what we are discussing isn't easy. And I also know that we all have body limitations, whether we believe it or not. I know a beautiful-bodied woman, a petite size 4, who won't go to the beach or even be caught dead near a pool. She calls herself "skinny fat," because although she loves her figure in clothes, she feels too flabby to take them off in public.

There are millions of "skinny fat" women hiding their bodies because they jiggle a bit here and there. Some of them tell me that they feel even more pressure to look amazing in a swimsuit because of how good they look in clothes. "Everyone tells me how incredible my figure is," one woman in particular shared with me. "They have no idea that underneath my tight jeans and padded bra, I have cellulite, sagging boobs, and a flabby belly. I'm not about to ruin my image with reality." These thin but unfit women avoid doing things just as many technically "overweight" women do because they're not yet in "good shape." How sad is that? There's a good probability that this woman (and the many like her) will never be any smaller or firmer than she is now, so what's she waiting for?

Women aren't the only ones with body image problems. It's also true for men.

"I'd love to read a book on body image," a man named Tom said to me the other day.

"Really?" I asked. "I thought my readership would be mostly women."

"That's what women think," he said, "but men have issues with their body, too."

This struck me as kind of funny initially. Not that I didn't think he was right, but this man was *really* cute. Big blue eyes, long lashes, beautiful skin, a thick head of dark wavy hair, with a fit, strong-looking body—just my type, actually.

"I don't know what you're writing about in your book," he continued, "but I've had insecurities my whole life, and I don't think they're much different than what women deal with."

Hmm. Now I was intrigued. "What do you feel insecure about?" I asked.

"For starters, I'm only five-six, and there were plenty of women through the years who wouldn't date me just because I'm short."

We had been sitting down, so I hadn't noticed his height, but I had to admit that I'm usually attracted to taller men. I felt a tinge of guilt suddenly, and a flood of compassion.

I didn't want to tell him that I had just read a study that explained that tall men, on average, earn more money in the workplace than short men. People, it seems (and not just women), view a man as more powerful, and thus a better leader, if he's tall.

In so many insidious ways our body is working for us or against us, based on our beliefs as well as the collective belief of the general public. Tall might be great for a man, but I know several tall women who have experienced ridicule throughout their lives for being "too tall." In an effort not to stand out so much, they start frumping their shoulders forward and looking down at the ground. Tall is beautiful in women, but many women report that being "too tall," whatever height that is for them, can be a liability.

Tom went on to tell me about other issues he's had in the past—things he's fixed—like being a bit overweight, having several large moles removed, and getting caps on his teeth. He was a great guy, and had been in a happy relationship for over a year, so I left our talk feeling good about his particular situation, but it got me thinking.

There are some things in life we cannot change. Our height, for one, and also things like the length of our fingers, the shape of our feet, the size of our bones, and the width of our hips or rib cage. A lot of other areas these days can be altered—our teeth, our hair color, the shape of our noses, our lips, our breasts, our fat content, and so on. But some of those changes can be expensive, painful, time-consuming, and even potentially dangerous—especially in the case of plastic surgery. I think most of our problems come when we feel helpless to change the things we do not love about ourselves, and give up.

We would all do well to learn the Serenity Prayer, which has been attributed to Reinhold Niebuhr. You've heard it before; part of it goes like this: *"God grant me the serenity to accept the things I cannot change / courage to change the things I can / and wisdom to know the difference."*

I especially like the part about accepting the things we cannot change. But here's the challenge: The things we cannot change about our bodies, when looked at, often bring up bad feelings or memories about things we cannot (or haven't been able to) change in our lives. And those same things can also affect our ability to go for our dreams.

Yes, our bodies have some real limitations, and we must accept them, but this doesn't mean we can't pursue some aspect of what we love. When we take our limitations out of the equation, suddenly many options become possible.

Learning to accept your body as is and choosing to be healthy and fit regardless of your limitations happens one awareness at a time, one action at a time. I had to start somewhere, and for me, it

all started with taking a small action. Small actions, when added together, make for big changes. Once you've answered—really
answered—the questions in this chapter (yes, I'm assuming a few of
you have rushed or skipped them altogether—so go back and do
them, okay?), then you will be ready to face the excuses you use to
keep those beliefs in place.

That's easier said than done, but that's why you're here. . . .

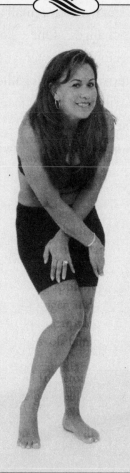

KRIS

Height: 5'4" • Weight: 146 pounds • Age: 39

Body Trap: *My feelings toward my body are dependent on how well I'm taking care of myself, and that's always inconsistent.*

Body Reality: *In clothes, I know how to hide my lumps and bumps. But in this, I feel exposed. It's hard to accept myself.*

Body Thoughts: *Men think I'm sexy, women think I should be smaller.*

CHAPTER 4

How Does My Body Hold Me Back?

I t's late, and I've just come home from a fourteen-hour day at
the *Starting Over* house. Exhausted and hungry, I kick off
my shoes and head to the kitchen. These are the nights when
I dream about having a loving husband waiting for me at home.
He'd meet me at the door and have a scrumptious meal on the stove
(because my fantasy includes a man who loves to feed me). Together, we'd eat, talk about our exciting days, and watch some
funny yet thought-provoking movie before snuggling into bed.

Humph. Maybe I'll treat myself to a plate of thick, sugary cinnamon toast tonight. *I'll get to the gym bright and early in the morning,*
I rationalize, *so I'll work it off then.* I only munched on a salmon
salad with greens all day, so I need some comfort food. That's all I
want right about now, except for that hunky husband.

I open the refrigerator. No bread. I've been so busy that I haven't been to the market in days. Darn it. Instead, I sit down with a boring bowl of plain oatmeal and riffle through the mail. Oh goody—a handwritten card. I wonder who has sent me a note?

"Join us for the last rays of summer, and bring your suit!" reads the cheery card, sent by a producer friend of mine. It's illustrated with a cartoon girl in a pink bikini, lounging on a floating mattress with a martini in her hand.

Oh no . . . not a pool party! A "Hollywood" pool party, no less. I've managed to make it through almost the entire summer dodging these soirees, without so much as putting a toe in a pool with others present, and I'm not about to start now! Frightening visions of attempting to get into my ten-year-old, partially faded black one-piece swimsuit flash before me. I can see it now: I'll be trying to hide my body all day long, while tanned bikini-clad women— swimsuit babes—frolic and sashay back and forth, free as flamingos.

There's no way I'm up for going to this swanky pool party in a swimsuit! Not even a remote possibility. If I can't get away with wearing a substantial, non-form-fitting summer dress, then count me out! This is Los Angeles, California, people. There are no other middle-aged women from the Midwest at these events. And that includes barbecues or picnics or any other happening where potential stripping of clothes is on the itinerary. RSVP: Rhonda Britten will not be attending, thank you very much.

I have been refusing to buy a new swimsuit for a long time now, which is why mine is ten years old. Not that I haven't given it the good old college try. It's just that each time I enter the store, I feel like I am gaining weight from the second I walk in, to the time I actually try something on. It's just pointless. I could blame it on the evil lighting, or their doubly evil mirrors (what kind of conspiracy is at work here?), but ignoring the issue is easier. Besides, I've convinced myself that I can only wear suits that are one-piece, cut under my breasts, and have a skirt, which are even harder to find than "normal" one-pieces. But I like the cut of these empire-waisted suits because they result in NO clingage. When nothing clings, I can relax a little more. But of course, I still have to wrap a towel around my waist, just to be safe.

I feel exposed in a swimsuit and that feeling of exposure can lower my self-esteem at a moment's notice, if I let it. And until now, I have been letting it. I don't think I am the only one.

Let's talk straight: If you didn't have to deal with your body, would you? I know a lot of people who go to great strides to avoid looking in the mirror, especially when it comes to seeing what's below their neck. They don't want to face their body. "I want to be healthy!" they say, but they do little to support that goal. And, even when they do, their efforts are short-lived because their negative habits are so ingrained.

"*I couldn't possibly wear that!*" becomes our immediate response—our total truth—and we'll cling to this belief with all our might. When someone suggests that you wear a bikini to the Saturday night pool party at the neighbor's house (after you've worn a one-piece for the last twenty years), it sounds ridiculous, and feels impossible. For many of us, changing our body (let alone our bathing suit) feels too hard—out of reach of what we can accomplish with our limited time, energy, and discipline. Maybe we have even tried, but the results, if we had any, weren't worth the Herculean efforts. And really, if we do hit our desired weight, as some of us have in the past, we'll only find other things to fret about (our hips, thighs, or our bellies), so never mind. We talk ourselves out of even trying, thinking any effort will never be enough . . . and this is how another year disappears without any changes. Except self-defeating ones.

Finding Our Comfort Zones

When Summer entered the *Starting Over* house, she refused to put on her bathing suit, even though night after night the ladies lounged in and around the hot tub. Bethany never wore anything that would reveal her calves, let alone her ankles. Christie had a difficult time baring her arms due to, in her words, her botched surgery. Here I was, helping them through their issues, all the while concealing my tummy behind flowing blouses, tailored jackets, and an empire-waisted bathing suit.

Staring at the invite, the question becomes: How long can I avoid pool parties and swimsuits, seeing as how I live in Los Angeles and coach women on loving themselves, no less? You can be assured I am not content to hide myself for the rest of my life. I'm also realistic, however, and I don't expect myself to be a spontaneous miracle worker. While I've seen and helped facilitate radical change in my clients' lives in short periods of time, I'm also choosing to be kind and patient with myself. I'm a working woman with a very full plate (pun intended), and I'm interested in making changes that will last over time. I don't mean to sound like I'm letting myself off the hook, and neither should you, but let's start off with the steps we can handle, the steps that will work and become the foundation for further action.

In my metaphoric version of doing the "doggy paddle" before learning the "butterfly" stroke, I have started facing my swimsuit fears by going to hotel pools while I'm traveling on the road. Easier, I decided, than starting by swimming at Hollywood pool parties. I put on my old one-piece suit, take off all of my makeup, and then cover my head with a big, floppy hat. Even if you were looking straight at me and thinking, "Oh goodness, that woman should never wear that," you'd *never* recognize me! I look like just another middle-aged woman from the Midwest, not someone trying to be a twenty-something pool babe.

In order to practice accepting my body and pushing past my comfort zone, I swim for a little while and then lay out a bit, feeling the gentle breeze blow over my body. When most of the water has evaporated and the sun once again feels hot on my skin, I walk to the side of the pool—less timidly this time than last—jump in, and swim some more. *You know, it feels good moving around like this,* I think to myself, with the warmth of the sun on my back and the water pressure against my face. I see something shiny and dive toward the silvery object at the bottom of the pool. For just a second, I feel like a kid again and pretend that I'm hunting for buried treasure. I stop and blow bubbles toward the surface and watch as the sun streams through the water and makes everything glisten. It's beautiful down here. I forgot how much fun swimming is! When, exactly, did swimming stop being about fun and get so entangled with feelings of fear and self-loathing? I'm transported to little-kid memories, and I'm remarkably free from worries of who sees me, or who thinks what about any of my parts. This is the freedom I want. This is the life I desire. This is a shift in the right direction. Maybe by throwing myself in the deep end (literally and figuratively), I'm demystifying the process. I make a mental note to try this with my clients.

Celebrating the Wins

I want you to get over your body and get on with your life, just like me. There are, of course, different ways to do that. You have to decide which approach is right for you, and that's the beauty of this process. There is no one "right" way to find your freedom. The point of this story is not to convince you that you must buy a bikini and attend parties that scare you. On the contrary, I don't know when I'll ever go to a pool party in a swimsuit that doesn't come with a matching skirt. What's important, though, is that I let go of trying to cover up that these parties bother me, and come to decisions I can live with about what I am willing to wear and with whom. Right now, I'm happy—make that *elated*—to even be swimming again. That, believe me, is a miracle, and it may be enough to make me smile for the rest of my life. Maybe, after months or years of swimming at home and around hotel pool strangers, I may be ready for the next phase: swimming with friends. We'll see. I have no problem with you having some limitations in your life, as long as you know what they are and can live with them happily. We can't do it all and be all things if we don't face the excuses we're using.

That's the point. I might not be perfectly healed about my body issues and I may not be fearless every minute in every situation, but I consistently make an effort to face, and break, my excuses. Still, there are times when I rely on my excuses. Picture this: I've got my short shorts on. I'm in hiking boots. I've just walked a treacherous trail. I've recently gone white-water rafting, and just the thought of it makes me feel strong and on top of the world. But what do I do when a hot man walks into the room? I'd like to say that I continue feeling fantastic—which has been the case on occasion. But it's also true that sometimes, even after all of my effort and recent heroics, it's not good enough. The excuses that I thought I had laid to rest all of a sudden become very loud again. The thought of this gorgeous man holding my hand or touching me brings up all of my body challenges. So I turn away. I hide in the back of the room or announce that I've got to leave for a meeting when really, I go straight home and watch TV, curled up in a ball on the couch.

Sometimes we're just cruising through our life and then something jars us out of our complacency. You get the invite to your twenty-year high school reunion. The man of your dreams wants to take you on a trip to the islands. You get the job you've always wished for but never thought would come your way. Even if you're a big success in your career or family, once you have to go back to your past, or experience a new uncomfortable situation that asks you to stretch beyond your comfort zone, your issues come flying back up to the surface and you want to run for the hills.

The reunion, the man, the promotion, the adventure of a lifetime, can all be stopped cold by your "can'ts." I can't see these people, I can't date that man, I can't take that job—*I can't because I'm not ready*.

For others, negative thoughts about their body are stirred up when it feels like their life is going down the tubes. Their body becomes just one more thing to add to their long list of complaints. Until they lost their job, their mate, or their health, they ignored their body. I mean, didn't they have a mate, a job, and their health when their body wasn't at its best? *What's the big deal; it works, doesn't it?* But then one day, it doesn't work, and the body they've been ignoring rears its head.

Remember my search for the perfect Emmy dress? I waited until the last minute to find it. Why? Because I wanted to avoid being disappointed one more time because of my body. And heck, I'm *so* busy. What a perfect excuse! How could I have the time to fix my body, let alone find the time to find a dress to hide my parts if I'm so busy? *Maybe I should just skip the whole Emmy thing*, I thought. Trust me, that went through my head. More than once.

Vanessa's body image also held her back. A client of mine in the *Starting Over* house, she attracted some of the strongest fan mail of any woman. Yes, you could say that Vanessa was popular because she's beautiful and, as a world-class athlete who had been sure to head to the Olympics as a gymnast, she was already known and loved by a legion of fans that had followed her career for years. But I think the single biggest draw about Vanessa was that she was publicly sabotaging her body (and her success) since giving up her Olympic dreams, through eating brownies and cakes when she wanted to cry, candy and bread when she felt ugly, and anything else that could fill her "hole" when she thought about the fateful day when she "messed up" during her Olympic trials.

Americans loved Vanessa because they could relate to her. Women sitting at home sabotaging their own bodies would root for her because she was doing what they were doing—and she was doing it in front of everyone . . . on TV! Fans secretly said to themselves: *If she can't stay thin and healthy and strong, how can I?* So, they sat at home, hoping and praying that Vanessa's courage would inspire their own.

Eventually Vanessa came to see that if she kept herself out of shape, she couldn't very well be a gymnast or ever think about trying out for the Olympics again. If she didn't try, she couldn't fail. As long as she was stuck feeling bad about herself, she would stay stuck and avoid any pressure from loved ones and strangers to achieve. Vanessa, therefore, had the perfect excuse for why she didn't have to put herself out there. Everyone knows you can't be fat and be a winning gymnast at the same time. It's just not possible. So, Vanessa could avoid her dreams and stay in her fear and it wouldn't even be her fault. Her body would be the one to blame. It was the ultimate excuse, even though in her mind, it's the one thing she *should* be able to control.

For many people, control plays a key role. It sounds like this: *I should be able to control my body, and if I can't, there's no point in fighting it. I'm just too stupid, too lazy, too selfish, too broken to do anything different.*

You and I know that isn't true. What are your excuses?

Your Exercise

What will stay the same in your life if you keep on hiding? What do you tell yourself you can't do because of your body? Go on. Let it out.

My body holds me back from doing . . .

Because of my body, I do not . . .

If my body were different, I would have the courage to . . .

Excuses let you off the hook (and excuse you) from living your potential, and that includes accepting your body and loving it fully. So listen to your words. Excuses are hidden within your complaints. What do you complain about? We all complain. I listen to women from all across the country, and here are some of the most common complaints I hear when it comes to taking charge of their body. You might want to make a check mark next to, or highlight, those that ring true for you.

I'm too busy; It's my metabolism; It's my genes; I'm on a seven-year pity party (and the party's over); My whole family is big; I'm too young to worry about that; I've got no motivation; I have a bad body type; I'm lazy; I eat too much; I'm too tired; I've got a wide waist; I'm pregnant; I hurt my hip in college and haven't been able to work out since; I like to eat a lot; I don't get enough exercise; I will never look like I did in my twenties, so why bother; I'll always look bad; It's impossible to have a flat stomach because I'm short-waisted; I'm too old; I'm sick; I gave birth to four kids; I have a bad knee; I'm too young to worry about it; I'm a stay-at-home-mom; Why improve my body when my husband wouldn't notice anyway; I've got big bones; I am hypothyroid; I'm menopausal; I just love food . . .

Just Like Everyone Else

The women you see throughout these pages were part of a group of forty-five women who came together to expose their bodies in front of a camera lens for the sake of demystifying the female body. They filled out a detailed questionnaire about how they treated their bodies and how they felt about their bodies, including how they felt about wearing tight black shorts and a black sports bra. For many, it was one of the most difficult things they had ever done. For some, it was a walk in the park. But everyone, at one time or another, had used their body as an excuse.

What events did these women avoid because of their body? Believe it or not, the Academy Awards were on the list—twice! Isn't that amazing? Millions of people in hundreds of countries dream of being able to walk down that most coveted of red carpets, and these ladies were willing to miss out on that experience so they could hide the way they looked! Three twenty-year high school reunions also made the list, as well as numerous vacations in the tropics, pool parties, dating, weddings, intimacy (in general), birthday parties, and so much more. Look at what people miss out on in life all because of the negative feelings they have about their bodies . . . some of the most celebratory events belonging to the human experience.

If you believe that you can't ever take control of your health, you won't. If you believe you don't have time for exercise, you will be right. If you believe your genes are more powerful than proper nutrition, you will do anything to prove your point. It's almost as if people need to believe their excuses, because in some weird way, being "right" is their barometer for success. And making the "right" decisions proves our value in a world that applauds success over truth.

Being right somehow convinces you that all the decisions you have made have been okay. Coming clean about the excuses you're using puts your entire past at risk for being plain ol' wrong. It makes sense that if you don't feel that you are thin enough, you really believe you aren't. It doesn't matter what I say. I can't convince you— just like you wouldn't be able to convince me that I'd look good in a bikini. Excuses *feel* real, even when you logically know you are making them up to avoid change.

We use our body as the ultimate excuse to get out of just about everything. You don't have to dance with the cute groomsmen at your sister's wedding if you feel like a pig in your bridesmaid dress. You don't have to date if you feel unattractive. You don't have to work hard to get that promotion if you believe overweight people are discriminated against in your work environment. *It's never your fault.* Your genes aren't your fault. Having three kids isn't your fault. Being broke isn't your fault either.

People use excuses because excuses work. I've used them with stellar results. If I don't call my best friend Marta on her excuses, she won't call me on mine. It's the silent agreement among friends. For many women, it's a condition of friendship.

Your Exercise

Following is a photo of my body. I've drawn circles around areas I've used as an excuse. For instance, my upper arms are circled because they jiggle and I use them as an excuse for why I don't wear tank tops or sleeveless dresses. This excuse seems perfectly logical to me, until I see a woman who is larger than me wearing something sleeveless and looking fabulous. I experience a twinge of jealousy about how free she is to express herself. Immediately I want to make up a story about her to validate my long sleeves in 90-degree heat. I will go on about her loneliness, frustrating career, and true unhappiness. I mean, in my world, you can't possibly be totally happy if you don't have thin upper arms.

It is in the midst of my storytelling that I realize I am talking about me and not her. My true happiness, once again, is compromised by my thinking. I am the one frustrated with aspects of my career, and I am the one who is lonely. I don't want to face those problems, so instead I make it about my "fat" arms. In that moment, I'm grasping for hope. The hope of thin arms seduces me into reading the latest fitness book and devouring magazine articles aimed at the same. Somewhere in the sickness of my mind, I believe that thin arms are the secret to happiness. All my problems will be solved if I have the discipline to change my arms and therefore my life. It's no wonder I manifested coaching a woman who nearly mutilated hers.

The hard truth is that my arms are not stopping me. They are merely a distraction.

What excuses do you tell yourself and the world around you? What parts of your body give you permission to hide behind your excuses? Find a picture of yourself, or feel free to use mine below. Grab a thick black marker, and start circling the body parts that stop you from living a life of freedom, and write down what you refuse to do because of those body parts.

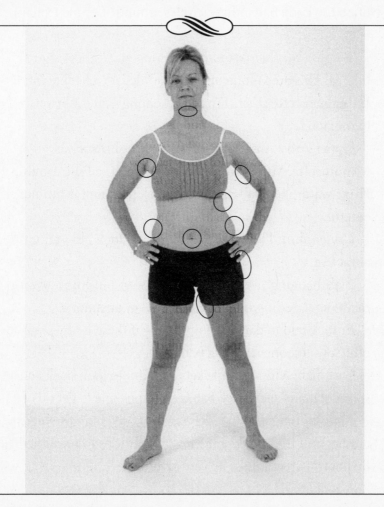

Just look at all the things your body stops you from doing. Is this reality okay with you? Do you want to be able to do more of what you love, or is your limited life adequate? What if I told you that excuses are no longer acceptable if you want to learn to accept your body? Just like me and my jiggly arms and bulging tummy, excuses have prevented me from whipping on my bathing suit and joining in the fun. I refuse to let my body stop me anymore.

Notice the body parts I have circles around? Let me explain.

Thighs: No thigh-exposing bathing suits, short shorts, bikinis. This area is one of my "thin" decade checkpoints. If thighs rub together, I'm not fit enough and, obviously to me, too fat.

Upper arms: Absolutely no sleeveless shirts. Ever.

Stomach: Must camouflage stomach at all times. Huge wardrobe challenge. I just look pregnant if I'm not careful.

Under chin: Double chin makes me look old and unattractive.

Flab hanging over my pants: No sexy hip huggers for me. Forget getting undressed in front of anyone.

Butt: Afraid to dance, jump, or jog if there is any possibility of someone standing behind me.

Back flab: Must wear jackets if I want to look sleek and slimmer than I feel. Back flab feels impossible to get rid of.

Flab coming out on the sides of my bra: Strategic clothes and the perfect bra are my solutions to minimize this horrid area. I must be very careful.

That was the old Rhonda. The new Rhonda refuses to let her body stop her anymore. Sure, I might have to take one step at a time, but I am moving forward no matter what my body looks like. I urge you to give up your excuses for why you aren't doing something. Either decide that it's not really important to you and stop expecting yourself to do it (find peace with the situation) or make a commitment to take one step toward that thing you fear—today.

For me, putting on a bathing suit still brings up pain and embarrassment, but instead of letting those feelings stop me, I use them to propel me forward. Last week I finally did attend one of those pool parties for a friend's birthday party and yes, at first, I felt ugly and fat. But then I decided to take back my body, celebrate myself, and focus on the risk I was taking. Are you willing to do the same? I dare you to drag out your faded black ten-year-old suit and jump into the deep end without looking back. No one laughed at me, by the way—at least not as far as I know—and in this case, it doesn't matter. What does matter is that in that moment, I was proud to be me.

Ask yourself: Are you proud to be you, or are you too busy wishing you were somebody else?

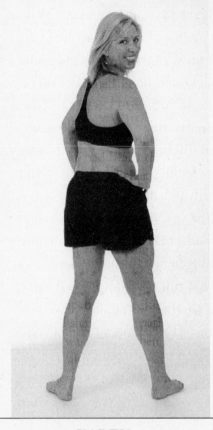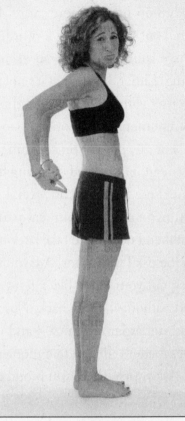

KAREN

Height: 5'7"

Weight: 160 pounds

Age: 39

Body Thoughts: *I've never been comfortable in my body. Something is always wrong.*

Body Weight: *I am always five to ten pounds heavier than I wish I could be.*

MARIA

Height: 5'6"

Weight: 120 pounds

Age: 26

Body Motto: *My body is unique to me. No one has my same scars or birthmarks.*

Body Complaint: *My body has the flattest butt in the world.*

CHAPTER 5

Who Am I Comparing Myself To?

J ust like the women in the *Starting Over* house, I have had to face the reasons I've hated my body, or different parts of it. Most women, I've found, don't readily admit to hating their whole body, but without much prompting, they'll quickly admit to hating one or more of the big three: the stomach, thighs, or butt.

"Does my butt look like her butt?" I whispered to my best friend Marta, pointing to the butt of a lady leaning over the counter at our favorite coffee shop. I knew that wasn't an enlightened question, but I couldn't help myself. I had been working out for about six months and was sure my butt had not changed an iota. I was secretly hoping I was wrong, but had to know the truth.

Marta looked at me as she always does when I'm feeling insecure, with a mixture of compassion and resignation. "Don't worry,"

I said, as I checked out the lay of the land. "I won't blame the messenger. Are you in?"

Marta nodded her head while rolling her eyes. I ignored her obvious distaste for the task, and continued on my mission. "Okay, I'll walk up to the counter and ask for change for the meter, while you compare us, okay? I want to know all of the facts. Is my butt bigger, smaller, wider, thinner, higher, or lower than hers?"

With that, I strolled up to the counter and leaned in, careful to stand in the same position as the woman (and generally make a butt of myself), before casually walking back to our table.

"So?" I asked, as soon as we were both seated. "How did I measure up?"

"Rhonda, your butt is definitely smaller," Marta assured me. "I've been telling you that you've lost inches. Why won't you believe me?"

Why would I choose not to believe my best friend, who in all our years of friendship has never so much as told me a white lie? Because, no matter how hard I work on my body, no matter how much I appreciate it for all it has done for me, there is that tiny piece of me that can't, or won't, believe that my body is enough as it is. I know intellectually that my body complaints are not really about my body—I know they're only the symptom of my fear that I will always be alone, that no one could really love me. Why, then, does all this awareness and good information do diddly-squat for me when I'm faced with trying to see the good where my body is concerned? Can I ever really learn to love myself?

Scared of the Truth

Comparing my body to another woman's is almost the worst thing I can do when it comes to healing my body image. It's a bad habit that I'm only just now shaking. For good reason: No matter how many times I look in the mirror, I feel that I have no perspective of what I really look like. Sometimes I feel like the image staring back at me is an optical illusion. I think I look one way, but when someone like Marta points out a comparable body, I am shocked. According to her, I always look better than I think I do. And when I am comparing my body to another, I'm always expecting the worst (and then, of course, I'm unable to accept the truth). I want to believe the better news, I really do. I am just scared. Scared of being duped. Scared of embracing a body that I might not have. (I mean, what if Marta's eyesight is faulty, or she just thinks I look better than I do because she loves me?) I'm scared of looking like a fool.

Do you ever feel the same? Do you look at other women's bodies and compare theirs to yours, hoping upon hope that yours is better? Do you ever befriend people because they have the body you want, and you pray that some of that good fortune will rub off by association? Or worse, do you ever make friends with people who have "worse" bodies than you do, just to make yourself feel better about your own situation? What about love? Do your dates or mates have, on average, bodies that are considered better or worse than yours? Do you have to be the pretty one, or are you okay if you feel your partner is better-looking? I know comparing myself to others isn't an evolved mind-set, but sometimes I just need to know. Regardless of my good intentions, there are times when my fears are still running the show.

You'd think that sisters and best friends would be excluded from the competition of comparing. Au contraire. Marta is not immune to my insatiable desire to win. But we don't call it competition. We call it friendship.

Marta and I can get into long dissertations on the ifs, ands, and buts of our butts. We kvetch about the need for a long-sleeved dress, even if it's a hot and humid summer day. We discuss why it's better to buy a larger pant size so they don't ride up and give us what Andy Paige calls the "smile across our crotch." We shop together, making sure we examine each other from all sides while also checking out the girl trying on the same dress in order to be sure we look better than she does. Then we eat dessert together, ruminating on how it's virtually impossible for us "normal" folks to have a tight, firm body. We confess to each other about how afraid we are of getting old and wonder if our bodies will even have a chance during menopause. If Jamie Lee Curtis—hard body of hard bodies in her prime— couldn't keep her weight down after "the change," what hope do we really have? What will happen to us? How will we successfully compete—for men, compliments, adoration, the best jobs, the best clothes—for anything?

That's what friends are for, right? To see the importance of this issue, to empathize with us, agree with us, and ultimately stay the same weight as us. You know, the old misery-loves-company arrangement? A silent contract with no winners. That's how it was with Marta and me. We had a great arrangement. Until the day she changed the rules.

"Betrayed" by a Friend

Marta and I had been talking about our body imperfections for years. Body disappointment is one of the things we have in common—one of our unwritten, sisterly, best-friends-for-life bonds. But secretly, I knew I couldn't complain as much as Marta because I was always smaller than her.

At five feet six inches, with a small frame (according to the health gurus and their weight charts), I should weigh between 120 and 125 pounds. During my divorce, I was at my heaviest weight, topping out at a whopping 160. Then I lost a little, and for most of the last ten years, my weight stuck at about 150 pounds, regardless of what diet or exercise plan I tried. Nothing seemed to nudge the scale down any lower.

Marta, unlike me, has large bones, and shares my height. We look eye to eye, but her weight has always been higher than mine—as it should be, what with those big bones and all. Everyone knows that bones are heavy, and bigger ones, heavier still. Even so, I've never thought of Marta as heavy. "I have big bones, which weigh more," she'd tell me. "And football shoulders." Okay. Sounded rational enough to me. If that's her body type, I reasoned, which she should know, who am I to disagree?

So that's the way it went. For years. I accepted that Marta would always be bigger than me. I would always be the winner of the "Who Is the Thinner Friend?" contest. Nothing more than factual science at work here—like how Jupiter looms many times larger than the earth, or how rocks weigh more than feathers—right?

Right. Until, that is, Marta joined Weight Watchers.

Competition is an ego-based thing, but sometimes it's the only thing that gets you off the couch. Marta did the unthinkable. She lost forty pounds in eighteen months! Sure, she would give me the updates about her food struggles and victories during her weight loss, but I was living in Colorado and Chicago, so I didn't actually set my eyes on her new frame until she was down to her goal weight of 139 pounds. I rang the doorbell of her environmentally friendly house in Los Angeles, and nothing could have prepared me to see the new Marta.

Marta was thin. But not the kind of thin that happens when you starve yourself and lose a ton of weight in too short of a time period. No. She was healthy thin. Glowing thin. Happy thin. After a year and a half of practicing better eating habits, my large-boned friend was smaller than I was! Her weight, her frame, her *everything* was smaller. Was it possible that even her bones had shrunk? All I knew was that I was no longer Lucy Ricardo and she, my Ethel Mertz. It was the other way around. I felt gargantuan.

I felt betrayed.

My mind raced to process the change. How had I missed the cues? The signs? The obvious? How could I have been so asleep at the wheel? Marta had told me how she was eating a huge salad every day for lunch and had even turned to asking me about my vegetable intake (maybe that's when I started tuning her out). She would tell me how she had lost another pound this week and would even go on and on about her daily walks—telling me how good it felt to get her heart pumping and her legs moving. But never once did I think it would add up to what was standing here before me. I didn't think it would actually work! But it had. As happy as I was for my dear friend (and I was), the fact remained that I now felt left out and left behind.

Marta didn't lose weight to become thin. She wasn't doing it to win the title of "Thin Friend." For her, it was never about the number on the scale giving her validation that she was good enough. Instead, Marta used the numbers as an external point of reference for how she was feeling about her body: The lower the number, the more she knew she was staying true to her commitment, feeling good about herself, and honoring her body. She used the numbers and the scale, not the other way around.

That was enlightening to me. I had never thought I could actually use the scale as a friend rather than a foe. I had no concept until that moment that a scale could merely be a fact-finding tool, a point of reference, like the texture of my skin or the size of my bra. It wasn't bad or good, it just was.

About the same time Marta had started Weight Watchers, I had begun working out in earnest. Not to lose weight, even though that was my secret wish, but under the premise to feel strong, flexible, and capable. I wanted to give up the competition and just learn to love what I had. I wanted my body to become a vehicle for pleasure, passion, and fun rather than something to hide or use as an excuse. If I wanted to kayak down a river, I wanted to paddle with the best of them. If I was invited to ski down the slopes, I didn't want my body to let me down. If a man went to hug me, I didn't want to contort my body into three different positions to avoid any real contact.

In those two years, I worked out at least three days a week, but I didn't lose a pound. In those same two years, Marta lost forty. What the heck?

Standing on Marta's doorstep, seeing her new thin frame for the first time, all my fears about my body came racing to the surface. I could feel all of my denial and anger, and nothing seemed okay anymore.

I wanted what Marta had. I wanted to be healthier *and* thinner. Somewhere inside of me, I was comparing myself to Marta because

I didn't want to be left behind. I wanted to be equal. I wanted to be enough. I wanted my friend to be as proud of me as I was of her. And in my mind, the new Marta couldn't possibly be.

I was scared to admit all of these conflicting feelings. How can you tell your friend, "I'm happy for you but I feel like a loser around you?" Because that is how I felt. I had translated being enough as, *I should be able to be just as thin, beautiful, and at peace with my body as my best friend.* My thoughts? *If you really loved me, you wouldn't change unless I was changing too!*

Of course, I knew in my heart that this wasn't the best approach. I knew my fear was clouding the reality that I was really happy for her. She had worked hard and it showed. I just felt like she had changed her life without me. I felt, once again, left behind (a theme in my life that I've experienced way too many times).

Intellectually, I understood that being healthier only translates to a longer, more productive, loving life. Isn't that what I *really* wanted? But emotionally, I was conflicted.

"How would you know any better when you and your sisters grew up competing for just about everything?" my dear friend pointed out. She was right. After Mom and Dad died, and probably even before that, my sisters Linda, Cindy, and I competed for affection, clothes, school supplies, and the last piece of chocolate cake. I never felt like enough of a winner in my own right, so unfortunately, I was bringing this competitive spirit into my friendship with Marta.

Family First

For all my complaining, I have to confess that I do love *some* things about my body. As an example, I love my skin. I pride myself on how soft it is, due in part to its virtually hairless quality. That's right, I have no hair on my arms, and little on my legs (my sisters don't even shave).

In the past, I used to advertise how soft my skin was, and yes, there have been times I've practically had a spitting contest with someone over whose skin was softer. I'd always won that competition until I accidentally rubbed up against my older sister Cindy's luxurious, silky skin. Without a doubt, her skin was softer than mine and I was not a happy camper. I mean, come on—she's four years older than me, an ex-smoker, and she buys the cheapest beauty products known to mankind, while I have never let a cigarette touch my lips, I know volumes about the best and latest beauty lotions and potions, and I'm younger than her. My sister, who clearly doesn't "deserve" better skin than me (according to my criteria), has me beat. That not only doesn't seem logical; it also doesn't seem fair.

Our pain ties into how we see ourselves and what we believe we're worthy of having. I hate it when I react like a petty, resentful, and jealous little kid (wanting what Cindy has, at the expense of our loving relationship). I want to stop justifying Cindy's right to have soft skin by pointing out how I may be "winning" in other areas. I only want to be genuinely happy for my sister—truly grateful that my sister has soft skin—without making it about me. I never want another person to fall victim to my low body confidence.

Maybe you indulge in similar thoughts from time to time. Since many of my conversations with my sisters and friends are centered around our bodies and who has what we want, I have a hard time believing this is only the case for my immediate environment. In fact, I see it daily in the *Starting Over* house. It's something to think about, and worth investigating. Perhaps your thought processes are more subtle, and your feelings whisper rather than yell, but it's worth knowing about just the same. Because unless you are completely honest about your feelings of jealousy, you will never move beyond your body issues. In reality, jealousy is a teacher giving you the next step on your path. It is showing you what needs to be healed.

Sisterly Love

Is there someone in your family that you compete with? Not only have I been spending my life competing with my sisters, but they also compete with me. When I started my self-care regime, my sisters didn't twiddle their thumbs. They jumped on the bandwagon, fearful *they* were getting left behind. Only recently have we admitted to each other that we have been secretly keeping track of one another's weight for decades. In fact, we've all been competing for the "Skinny Sister" title.

My younger sister, Linda, is usually the winner of the unofficial position because she is shorter, thinner, and more petite in general than my older sister, Cindy, and me. Linda hates it when I call her my "little sister," but that is what she has been for most of my life. Standing a tad more than five feet tall, weighing, on average, 110 pounds, she's the smallest in the family. There have been several instances when she's reached 120 pounds, but never for long. She's the one who joins Weight Watchers and reaches her goal weight within two weeks. It's sickening.

Cindy is five feet four inches tall and weighs around 125 pounds, give or take a pound or two. For decades, she has maintained that weight through two-hour daily hikes and eating at home more often than not. Controlling what goes into her mouth (and her family's) is a source of pride for Cindy and something I have always envied.

You can imagine how I have felt my entire life being the "biggest" in the family. In sister photos, I am always in the middle, not only because I am the middle girl, but because I think the pictures will be lopsided if I'm at either end. I realize I might be considered petite to some, but to my sisters, I am the "big one," and that has had an effect on my self-esteem.

I may not win a weight contest with my sisters, but one thing I have been working on is creating a new category—based more in a spirit of fun competition and healthy motivation: Who is the fittest? With my healthy lifestyle plan now integrated into my life, I am seeing results for my body like never before. My sisters are also seeing my results. Let's just say they are worried. So worried, in fact, that when we started to plan our next family vacation, at the beach, their health regimes accelerated to match mine.

Linda has started yoga classes, purchased a treadmill, and has been eating spinach salads. And if you knew Linda, you would understand that this is a shift of miraculous proportions. Linda is not known for her healthy food choices. In the past, her family's diet consisted largely of yogurt, cereal, and nachos. But times are a-changin'.

Cindy, who's always been the healthiest in the food department, stepped up her healthy habits by adding yoga, chiropractor visits, and bi-weekly Reiki massage. She's embracing activities that would have been considered "weird" to her just a few years ago.

Why the sudden change? Why compete with *me*? As Linda announced on one of our many calls, "I don't want to be the fat sister." We pretended to laugh, but in reality, we knew she was serious.

The Green-Eyed Giant

I see women come into the *Starting Over* house wrestling with these uncomfortable feelings of jealousy and competition. They want to see each other as "sisters," and often do (certainly more so as time goes by), but it's natural to compare and cut down another when feeling insecure. (It's not right, but it's human.) We have so much power, but we use it for the wrong things. We use it to abuse our bodies and hurt our hearts, all because we are afraid to deal with our feelings.

When I compare myself to another, it proves that I am not doing what I need to do to appreciate my body as it is. I don't need to wait for some future goal, like when I lose weight. Or when the man of my dreams loves all of me. I must appreciate my body, now. Right now.

Competition can either motivate you to change, or kill your sense of possibility.

When I'm feeling jealous, it means I'm not taking care of business—my business. I'm not taking responsibility for the plight of my body, the state of my life. Instead of changing my life, I am spending my time complaining about it. *If only I had her body*, I ponder, *my life would be perfect*. I know that isn't true, but when the green-eyed monster is running my life, it *feels* true.

Weight is a handy excuse. When we have too much of it, it literally holds us back. We move slower. We can't lift anything with ease. Our joints hurt and our muscles ache. It's as if our weight becomes a way to shield ourselves from the world. And when we can't do the things we want to do, we are jealous of those who can. We want to figure out a way, any way, to put them down so we can feel better about ourselves even for a moment.

Our jealousy feels so justified. To soothe the savage beast within, we splurge on the sixty-inch-monitor TV because we tell ourselves we deserve it. We want to reward ourselves after a hard day at work, so we drive to the grocery store to pick up that special treat so we can indulge in front of our favorite sitcom. But don't we deserve so much more? Don't we deserve to be in charge of our health, our weight, our bodies?

There are so many ways to heal a jealous heart, and I can speak to what I've seen work (and am experiencing myself). For starters, never underestimate the power of gratitude.

Your Body Is Your Friend

Compared to the past, I rarely beat myself up or call myself a "loser" when I feel like I've lost control over my weight. I have, finally, found a place of compassion for myself, which seems to have released a lot of the pressure I was feeling to "win the battle" over my body (and with other people). Ironically, I'm feeling better and lighter all the time—and I have more energy.

Ask yourself: What gives you permission to put yourself down and beat yourself up? Do you compare yourself with the latest movie star, a coworker who doesn't work out but has your dream body, or a past version of yourself? Or could just the mere fact that the body looking back at you in the mirror (if you look in the mirror) is not perfect or what you expect (or want) your body to be?

Today I want you to ask yourself if you are willing to love all of you—body included. In order to do that, you must give yourself an honest appraisal. Which parts of your body do you feel are the enemy? Perhaps your knees creak and your ankles crack, leaving you with too many aches and pains. Maybe your neck is showing your age, or your hands swell up every time you have your period. Don't worry. We'll do this together.

It's time to list all the ways in which your body hasn't been a friend to you. (The things we don't like about ourselves are usually the reasons we compare ourselves to others.) Let's start by naming the body parts that you'd like to change and why. I'll go first.

1. My knees are not my friends because they hurt all the time and they look ugly.
2. My hands are not my friends because my cuticles are always ragged and my fingers are short and stubby.
3. My stomach is not my friend because it has never been flat, no matter what I weigh, and a scar on my belly only makes it worse. The scar forms a pouch on my stomach that I can never get rid of. The scar makes me feel defeated about losing weight because no matter how thin I get, it will still be there. I will always have that scar; therefore, I will always be ugly.
4. My upper arms are not my friends because no matter how much I work out, they still sag.
5. My heart is not my friend because it jumps all over the place, making me feel insecure, unsure, and unsafe. I'm frequently left wondering if I'm about to have a heart attack.

Your Exercise

Get the idea? I want you to admit what bugs you about your body. It will help you realize which body parts give you permission to sabotage your good intentions. If you're like me and have a scar, you might be accustomed to using it as an excuse. For example, if I eat less ice cream, the scar will remain, so why not go ahead and have the mocha chip? My scar gives me permission to give up. How do your body parts do the same?

I will help you start by giving you some sentences to get the ball rolling. Just fill in the blanks and let whatever comes up be your answer.

1. My skin is not my friend because _wrinkles, dark circles, + zits_
2. My neck is not my friend because _____.
3. My chin is not my friend because ___blackheads___.
4. My mouth is not my friend because _____.
5. My forehead is not my friend because _blackheads___.
6. My breasts are not my friends because _they are starting to sag_.
7. My shoulders are not my friends because _____.
8. My stomach is not my friend because _its flabby and scarred_
9. My waist is not my friend because _its too wide_.
10. My hips are not my friends because _____.
11. My thighs are not my friends because _____.
12. My ankles are not my friends because _____.
13. My calves are not my friends because _____.
14. My toes are not my friends because _____.
15. My fingers are not my friends because _bad nails_.
16. My hands are not my friends because _age spots___.

17. My elbows are ~~not~~ my friends because _____.
18. My arms are ~~not~~ my friends because _____.
19. My butt is ~~not~~ my friend because _____.
20. My feet are ~~not~~ my friends because _____.

Now that you've gotten started, keep going. . . .

My _____ *is not my friend because* _____.
My _____ *is not my friend because* _____.
My _____ *is not my friend because* _____.
My _____ *is not my friend because* _____.
My _____ *is not my friend because* _____.
My _____ *is not my friend because* _____.
My _____ *is not my friend because* _____.
My _____ *is not my friend because* _____.
My _____ *is not my friend because* _____.
My _____ *is not my friend because* _____.

Thank you for being honest! I believe that we can only quit comparing ourselves when we are willing to embrace our body as it is. To change our body image, we must be brutally honest about what we really think. Not the nice version we tell our mothers or coworkers, but the real feelings we have about our body in the middle of the night after polishing off a pint of ice cream (or downing a fruit smoothie that has more fat grams than a classic pound cake). It's time to tell ourselves the truth, so that we can honestly face and overcome our fears.

How did it feel to admit your feelings for your entire being from head to toe?

Were you surprised at anything you said? Explain.

What body part made you feel most justified in feeling betrayed, hurt, or angry? *my belly - its my biggest problem area and its so hard to change*

If you could trade in one body part and only one, which one would it be? Why?
Belly -

As I discussed previously, we can trade in our cars for a better model. We can upgrade our kitchen cabinets and appliances. We can renovate our house. The one thing we cannot do is exchange our body for another one. We can have plastic surgery to transform some parts of ourselves, but there is no such thing as a full-body makeover for the average person, regardless of the reality shows that air. And truthfully, even the best cosmetic surgeons can't transplant cuticles or completely alter the genetics behind a pear-shaped appearance or funny-looking ankles.

In order to heal our body, we must heal our prejudices against it. It's the only way we will finally see the beauty of our body. We must be willing to name the enemy as a friend. We must look for the silver lining of the gray cloud. We must be willing to see the parts of our body we despise with love in our eyes. I didn't say that it would be easy, but it must be done. We must become grateful for what we have, no matter how we feel about it.

I want you to practice seeing your body through kind-hearted eyes. I want you to try to find something good about every body part that you just labeled, in your own way. I want you to figure out how you can turn around the negative chatter in your brain and attach something positive to say about every body part you're fortunate enough to have. (That's a hint. You really are fortunate to have all of them, in case you can't think of anything nice to say.) I want you to practice loving yourself.

Remember, facing your body helps you face yourself.

Let's try together, shall we? I'll go first.

1. My knees are my friends because they help me walk, run, jump, and move sideways, as well as forward and backward. They help me walk toward my work, which helps me be of service.

2. My hands are my friends because they help me communicate to the world through typing on a keyboard. People tell me that I talk with my hands through my gesturing, touching, and hugging—and that sounds like a positive.

3. My stomach is my friend because it reminds me that I am a woman who has experienced life. And I am grateful that it can absorb nutrients from my food and help convert them into energy.

4. My upper arms are my friends because they allow me to hug the people I love, reach out to new and old friends, and lift people up.

5. My heart is my friend because it reminds me to be gentle, to go slow, and to nurture myself.

As I search for the good inside what appears to be bad, I am giving myself a choice. My body isn't bad or good, it just is. I am the one who has been labeling it. And I have the power to label it whatever I want, no matter what appears "real" to the outside world.

Are you willing to see yourself differently and be appreciative and grateful for each of your body parts? I think you'll find that it's a lot of fun finally loving yourself.

Don't be surprised if this work seems difficult. When I gave this assignment to Bethany soon after she moved into the *Starting Over* house, she just stared at me like I was crazy. *"Like my body? Why would I do that?"* she asked. One of the greatest joys of my career was seeing Bethany eventually understand why, and actually embrace her figure.

Take your time. If you can't answer all of the questions below, complete what you can. Then come back and try again. If there are some questions that feel impossible to answer, leave them blank. These will be like small guideposts to point you in the direction of potential growth areas to come. Remember, when we can become grateful for our body parts, we will eventually become a friend to our body as a whole.

So, go ahead and begin. . . .

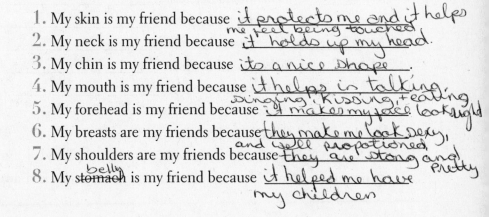

1. My skin is my friend because *it protects me and it helps me feel being touched*
2. My neck is my friend because *it holds up my head.*
3. My chin is my friend because *its a nice shape* .
4. My mouth is my friend because *it helps in talking, singing, kissing, + eating*
5. My forehead is my friend because *it makes my face look right*
6. My breasts are my friends because *they make me look sexy, and well proportioned,*
7. My shoulders are my friends because *they are strong and pretty*
8. My ~~stomach~~ belly is my friend because *it helped me have my children*

9. My waist is my friend because *it gives me a nice figure*

10. My hips are my friends because *they give me shape and*
   feel great when I dance.
11. My thighs are my friends because *they are strong*

12. My ankles are my friends because *they are strong + healthy*

13. My calves are my friends because _____.

14. My toes are my friends because *they are cute*.

15. My fingers are my friends because *they do so much*
   for me.
16. My hands are my friends because *touching*.

17. My elbows are my friends because *help my arms bend*

18. My arms are my friends because *reaching, hugging*
   stretching
19. My butt is my friend because *its sexy and strong*

20. My feet are my friends because *they let me walk*.

Keep going . . .

My _____ *is my friend because* _____.

My _____ *is my friend because* _____.

My _____ *is my friend because* _____.

My _____ *is my friend because* _____.

My _____ *is my friend because* _____.

My _____ *is my friend because* _____.

My _____ *is my friend because* _____.

My _____ *is my friend because* _____.

My _____ *is my friend because* _____.

My _____ *is my friend because* _____.

How does it feel to see your body as your friend?

What was the hardest body part to call friend?

Are you willing to believe what you just wrote down?

How could your life be different if your body was your BEST friend? Where could it take you? What could you do together? Who could you become? How could you love?

Ultimately, it's your choice to see your body as a friend or foe. When it's a friend, you will have no need to compare and compete with anything but your own good intentions. You will finally feel grateful for what you have and give up being angry at what you don't have. When it's a foe, you will continually look outside yourself to compare how you are doing because you have no internal compass, no sense of yourself.

When Bethany started this exercise, she had no idea how deep her dislike for her body ran, until I started asking her the same questions I'm asking you right now. She had a dickens of a time coming up with anything positive, besides naming the basic bodily functions. But that was a start.

What if your loyal, energetic, beautiful best friend of a body has been beside or inside of you for years, just waiting for you to give it some credit? Your body has worked hard at providing for you, caring for you, and loving you. Have you done the same for it?

I encourage you to decide today to practice loving compassion toward your body for the next twenty-four hours. Every time you see your reflection in a mirror or a windowpane, silently say, "Thank you."

Being willing to see your body in a positive light will help shift your attitude from being a victim of your body to being a friend to your body. It will help elevate the need to compare and compete with those around you, because you will know that you are enough. Then you will be on the path toward believing that you are worth loving. . . .

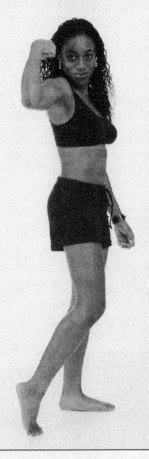

SADE

Height: 5'1½" • Weight: 110 pounds • Age: 25

Body Commitment: *I spent years not appreciating my body and decided one day to appreciate what I was given. I make sure I look in the mirror and love what I see, and that's why I am more confident today.*

CHAPTER 6

Can I Ever Really Love Myself?

Recently, my friend Marta and I were out to lunch, and she was convinced that a man at a nearby table was checking me out. I shrugged my shoulders and changed the subject. She changed it back.

"Why wouldn't you believe that man could be interested in you?" she demanded.

I tried to brush her off, but she insisted. I sat silently ashamed of what my answer would be. A tear rolled down my cheek, and she gently pressed her hand on mine and said, "Rhonda, don't do this to yourself. You are a beautiful woman. Once again you are doing to yourself what you did twenty years ago. You are not appreciating what you have." I knew she was right. Then came the final blow. "You don't want to be sitting here ten years from now and wishing you had the body you have now, do you? Follow your own advice. Don't set yourself up to live with regrets, Rhonda."

My Faded Past

What Marta was saying was true. Although I've nearly stopped comparing myself to people in restaurants and given up tracking my sisters' weight, there's still someone that I can't stop comparing myself to, no matter how many times I pray for a reprieve, or how often I counsel myself. Her name is Rhonda Britten, and she's from the past—she's my former self. Not so much the face or even the hair of my past self, but definitely the body I used to have . . . at eighteen, twenty-five, and thirty years old. I think being haunted by my "better body" is the worst of all setups. It keeps me living in the past, and sucks me into regret, where I continue to ache to be the way I once was.

My nieces Deena and Rachel live with me every summer during their college breaks. They work for me at the Fearless Living Institute, running errands, speaking to clients, and generally doing what needs to be done to keep my business, and my life, in order. Each summer they tell me during my workouts and trips to the health food store how beautiful I am. I thank them and do more sit-ups.

This past year, as Rachel was helping me prepare to move once again to Los Angeles for another season of *Starting Over*, we were rummaging through my closets and I found a pair of beat-up jeans shorts I used to wear back when I was her age. They were small. Smaller than I had remembered. Just looking at them, I knew I couldn't fit into them anymore, no matter how much I tried. But an idea came to me; maybe Rachel could? With that, I threw them over to Rachel and asked her to give them a try.

Rachel slipped off her baggy gym shorts and easily slipped into the jeans shorts I wore at nineteen. They fit her like a glove. As I stared in disbelief, tears started to flow. I took Rachel in front of the full-length mirror and stood next to her to compare my adult self to my nineteen-year-old niece wearing the shorts I wore at nineteen. Please understand, I adore my nieces as much as if they were my own children, so of course I was thrilled she could wear them. But on a whole other plane, I was devastated. In alternating between looking at her young body in my ripped and faded jeans shorts, and my chunky self in khaki shorts that were significantly larger, I felt like a blimp. That nineteen-year-old body seemed so far back in my past—so unreachable now.

I was torn between the memories of the body I had in my younger days, and the knowledge that age changes things. I'm a grown adult, with a very adult life, and I didn't want to be unrealistic. It's not like I was the only woman in the world who has gained a few pounds either. I didn't want to blow this out of proportion, and I didn't want to fall into the trap of giving an old pair of shorts too much of my power. But that didn't change the fact that I was sad. Sad for what I had lost—or gained, rather.

I knew somewhere inside of me that I had the potential to be happier in my body as an adult than I ever had in my youth. Back then, I used my body to get attention from others, specifically men. Thank goodness I grew to know better and value my mind and heart and my place in the world. There's no way I wanted to be nineteen years old again, but, oh, to have that body. The thought of it was so seductive.

At that moment, standing next to my niece, however, the possibility of attaining my past figure seemed incomprehensible. I knew I would never again be as tiny as my teenage niece. *How were my hips ever that small?* I wondered. *And how did mine get to be so wide today?* I couldn't blame the spread on having kids, because I've never received that pleasure. Did my hips—my very bones—expand two sizes from eating too many pieces of pie?

As Rachel threw off my shorts, I picked them up, determined to figure it out. I had to find out how far away this body was from all those years ago. While Rachel's back was turned, I escaped into the privacy of my bathroom. Taking off my khakis, I put both legs into the jeans shorts and yanked them up. They went up to my knees and stopped cold. *That's ridiculous*, I thought to myself. *I am not that fat. I am not that much bigger than my nieces, am I?* I bent down and pulled some more. I was determined to get them up, even if that meant only an inch or two more. With my next yank came a loud tear. I sat down on the toilet imagining what I must look like. I wanted to laugh, but instead, I cried. Again.

This time, however, I didn't cry for my lost body. Instead, I cried for all the years I wasted comparing myself to the past. Cried for all the times I told myself if I just tried harder I could get back my nineteen-year-old body. I cried because instead of appreciating what I had become, I'd been comparing myself to a faded memory of the past. One that didn't make me happy anyway.

Regret. It's a powerful emotion that has kept me stuck in a perpetual cycle of hating my body and then trying to make up for all the damage I have done to it—until now. I'm learning that my body is enough. Now I just have to figure out how to believe that it will be enough for someone else to love me. One step at a time, Rhonda.

The Naked Truth

As a single woman trying to date, when a man flirts with me, all I can think about is, *Then what?* I flirt back, we might exchange numbers, but what comes next? I mean, I know I can look good in clothes—he wouldn't be flirting with me if I didn't—but naked? I am a forty-five-year-old who desperately wants a relationship, yet I realize that if I have one, I will have to, in reality, become intimate at some point. And many men would prefer that to be sooner rather than later.

Starting to date and moving toward intimacy used to be a gradual process—often a slow build that would lead up to a steamy end. Nowadays, however, "hooking up" happens in the blink of an eye, and I'm not yet sure how to play this game. It seems to me like the dating world has become a place where checking out the mutual compatibility of libidos takes precedence over mutual respect, interests, and values. That's tough for a person like me, someone who has a difficult time being turned on without an emotional and intimate connection.

We've all experienced the internal conflict between our apprehension about our body, our fear of being alone, and our need to feel wanted. Those feelings can be easily jumbled together, leaving the lovelorn confused and frustrated. When that confusion ensues, we feel stuck, lonely, and afraid, which can lead to devastating results: staying in dissatisfying relationships, telling ourselves dating isn't worth it, or becoming a serial dater without experiencing a truly loving relationship.

As Marta was calling me out on my issues that day in the restaurant, I realized that my body confidence, or lack thereof, was standing in my way of experiencing love. Not just self-love, but also love from others—mates and friends. If I couldn't believe that a man was flirting with me, how would I ever believe someone wanted to make passionate love to me? Because "me" isn't Rhonda Britten, successful Life Coach. "Me" is my aging body, with sag, cellulite, and all. That "me" is harder to expose.

The Younger Man

It all happened innocently enough. Ted and I had been checking each other out for a few weeks—exchanging funny e-mails, finding ways to "accidentally" run into each other, and making sure our eyes met as we shared a laugh over a latte. During that time, I had rationalized in my mind that he probably figured I was thirty-eight. Most people do, even though I'm forty-five. Let's just say, I was banking on it. As we got to know each other, I figured he was about thirty-five. Great, I thought. That gives us a three-year age difference (using my thirty-eight as a fact and his thirty-five as a reality). But I was wrong.

I was introducing Ted to a producer who works with me on *Starting Over* when the two discovered they hailed from the same area of Chicago. "Do you know so-and-so?" went the conversation. I busied myself in paperwork while their small chat went on. Then the fatal question came: *"When did you graduate from high school?"* I pretended not to listen, but held my breath waiting for Ted's answer. "1993." WHAT? In 1993, I was in the midst of my depression and on the verge of getting divorced . . . and Ted was graduating from high school! I wanted to run out of the building, or scream, or throw up.

I tried to keep myself together. *Stay present Rhonda. Smile. Pretend you are okay with this devastating news.* I had never asked Ted how old he was because, truthfully, I didn't want to know. I wanted to keep the fantasy alive that this younger man could want me. But we weren't three years apart, like I had fantasized, but fifteen. Somehow those additional years added up to one word: Impossible.

Now that the truth was out, I felt old. Real old. Older than the hills, and much older than I had just a minute before. As I caught my breath, I flashed on a memory of seeing a photo of a happy Demi Moore wrapped around Ashton Kutcher, who, as you know, is fifteen years her junior. *But she is in shape.* I was screaming inside loud enough for myself to hear. *This isn't about age, it's about my body. Demi can have Ashton because she doesn't look her age. I do. Especially this minute. I look every bit forty-five. Who am I kidding?*

If I could have crawled into a hole and died, I would have. But we were in my office at the *Starting Over* house, with over a hundred employees within earshot. I was about to go on camera and change someone's life. I didn't have time to get philosophical; I had to use every bit of energy I had left to coach a woman into her greatness.

I excused myself from the room, ran to the bathroom, took a deep breath and walked back into my office knowing Ted would have to leave soon. He had just stopped by to say hi. I know what you're thinking. That means he did like me. I would have believed that, too, if 1993 wasn't a reality. But it was. And I knew I could no longer get past our age, or should I say the age of our bodies. Sure, he might want to flirt with me, but love me? That felt out of reach.

I had yet to truly embrace all of me, wrinkles, cellulite, and all, so embracing Ted's affection seemed an impossibility. Now, today, I know different.

Abandoned Again

When I found out that Ted was thirty, all I could think about was the age of the women I was competing with. They had to be in their twenties, mostly, with bodies of twenty-year-olds. Firm, tight, youthful bodies, a body I hadn't seen in twenty years. I'm almost too ashamed to admit that I thought so little of myself. But who can blame me? I've been rejected before. First, by my father and then, by my husband. One man killed himself in front of me while the other just got up and left.

Ten years before Ted, I was at a low point in my life, and my weight was at its highest. But my weight wasn't the real cause of my distress, it was only the symptom. Instead, it was my husband's rejection that seemed to be ruining my life. Allow me to backtrack.

Carl, my now ex-husband, and I had been having sexual issues. The issue was simple, really. He didn't want any. When it came to sleeping with me, Carl just wasn't interested in anything *but* sleep. I was in my mid-thirties and in love with my husband. I remember telling him that I had so much love for him, that finally, for the first time in my life, I felt that I had enough love to share with a child. I was ready to get pregnant. But I needed his help.

His "help" never came. So I gained weight. Not purposefully. It just happened. Or so it seemed. The pounds slowly crept on. Five pounds. Ten pounds. Twenty. Then thirty. Overall, I gained a quarter of my body size in twelve months.

At first I told myself I was gaining weight because I had read somewhere that a little extra weight increased your likelihood of becoming pregnant. But as the pounds increased, my self-esteem took a nosedive. I started to blame myself for our lackluster sex life. I remember looking in the mirror after a year of this and realizing no one would ever want me, not looking like this. *Who could blame my husband?* I thought. *I wouldn't want me either.* I remember thinking that if I just looked like my mother, then this wouldn't have to happen. She was beautiful no matter what was going on in her life, but not me. When my life was looking down, so were my looks.

To heap more humiliation on top of my fragile ego, when I was at my heaviest, I refused to purchase clothing that had to be zipped or buttoned shut. I became a fan of elastic waistbands. I wore flowing tops that hid my unsightly stomach. I was thirty-four years old and incredibly ashamed of my ever increasing plump form.

But no matter how many pounds I added, I refused to deal with Carl's rejection. In reality, I knew it wasn't his fault that I had put on weight. I was the one who refused to take charge of my body by eating right and exercising. I was the one who didn't want to deal with her marital woes. I was the one who didn't love herself enough.

Back then, the only thing I knew how to do was put my husband's needs before my own, just like my mother had done with my father. I was so afraid to lose him that compromise, or self neglect, seemed to be the only answer. I thought that was love. I see now that, in a weird way, I gained weight to save myself—from feeling rejection, from feeling loneliness, from confronting the problems I had long before our marriage. And the only way I knew how to save myself was to have my body say "no" for me.

My weight gave me full permission to say "no" to everyone. I was too embarrassed to go out. I was too ashamed to meet new people and take new risks. It forced me to be alone, unable to use my body for attention. Yet, in some miraculous way, it also gave me the time I needed to heal. This doesn't make rational sense, of course, but I hope you understand.

Gaining weight in and of itself isn't a bad thing when you can see it as a symptom of a deeper issue. And I do realize that all weight gain isn't psychological in nature. Yet like any symptom, any type of body dissatisfaction that goes on too long without being treated can become a debilitating disease for those who prefer to stay in the dark. My husband leaving was the best thing that ever happened to me. Of course I didn't know it at the time because I just felt ugly, fat, and repulsive. Now, I see it was the opening I needed to heal my life. It forced me to wake up to the fact that I had needed men to make me feel like I was sexy, beautiful, and enough rather than relying on my own sense of self. Without my husband to distract me, I got the wake-up call: *Rhonda, you can no longer wait for others to love you; you must love yourself.*

Much of our excess weight is caused by the shameful feelings we harbor about our past failures, family histories, and disappointments in ourselves. A form of protection on the one hand, and a route to self-punishment on the other, our weight keeps us trapped in a self-perpetuating state of self-hatred that lets us off the hook when it comes to the bigger issues. How can we find love, get married, or be all we can be when our body stands in our way? It's the perfect excuse, isn't it?

I don't think it's easy for anyone, including me, to talk about the negative effects our body image has had on our sexuality—it's humiliating and humbling. I so want to be more evolved than this, but find that when it comes to my body and intimacy, I feel vulnerable, scared, and emotionally naked. Without my negative body image to stop me, I could get hurt, be made a fool, or worse—I could fall madly, deeply in love.

History of Attraction

At an early age, I came to the conclusion that there were only so many boys around. Unless you were the prettiest or the thinnest or the most popular (which means you were the previous two), you didn't stand a chance with the most popular or best-looking boys. In many ways, times haven't changed all that much. For the most part, we're still haunted by the mythical image of Cinderella and the wicked stepsisters: We will finally "become special" if and only if we get recognized by our one and only. Our body becomes our calling card, and for many of us, that greatly limits our options—perceived or real.

Why the limitations? Because women, for the most part, still believe that a good mate is hard to find. The average woman wants a loving relationship so badly, but concedes her body will never be good enough to please, let alone keep, her soulmate. Thankfully some women aren't stopped by their bodies. In fact, their body is something that they have learned to embrace, love, and enjoy. The rest of us run around praying someone will finally make us feel safe enough to get undressed. It's almost as if we need permission before we will show off our assets, let alone reveal our hearts.

Settling for Less

The good news is that as we age, there is an opportunity to express our sexuality with greater freedom than we may have felt in our youth. Hopefully, we have become wise enough not to care if our breasts are sagging while making love. I mean, who doesn't feel sexier when they are loved? And hopefully, as we age, we have experienced love in our lives. We know what love is. We understand that beauty, even in our mates, is temporary, and that's okay. But even then, there are no guarantees that we won't get hurt.

My girlfriend just moved to the suburbs and meets regularly with the other moms in the neighborhood. When they get together, they talk, as women do, about their fears and concerns and hopes and dreams. Invariably, the conversation turns toward their husbands, and how difficult relationships can be. . . .

"My husband won't wash a dish to save his life," says one.

"I know what you mean! Mine won't either. But what bothers me more is how my husband throws his dirty clothes *everywhere*," says a second woman.

"That ain't nothing," says a third. "Mine just lost all of our savings in the stock market!"

"Yeah," says the fourth woman, "but it's better than getting a divorce, because if I ever left my husband, I'd have to get a boob job!"

My friend stopped here, ready to explain what the woman had meant, but I told her it wasn't necessary. I knew exactly what she was talking about, and so did her three friends. I know several women right now with one foot in their marriage and one foot out, yet they won't leave. Just the thought—the mere thought—of going to bed with another man is enough to stop them in their tracks. No matter how much he irritates you, your husband has seen you earn those sagging boobs with his children or with the passing of the years. He saw the reason for the sag and the stretch marks, and has to cut you some slack. You allow yourself some slack as well, knowing that he understands what you've been through. He's seen you build your business, or go through years of stress, and you gained those pounds together. You ate those pints of ice cream as a couple.

But with a new man? The birth of *his* kids didn't cause those stretch marks. He wasn't around when you were working all day and taking night classes in order to get your degree. He didn't see how much you ran to junk food to help you stay up. Chances are, he just left a woman with her own sags and stretch marks, and you're convinced that he's looking for a younger, more perfect model.

That younger, "perfect" model, well, she ain't me. My friend's conversation has been ringing in my brain as I make my way through the precarious world of dating. Just as body image has affected these women's relationships with their husbands, my ability to be comfortable in my body has determined my dating success and, in the past, sabotaged it. Because of that, dating can feel like a minefield of potential disaster. What chance do we have to satisfy our intimate sexual desires if we don't feel attractive enough to deserve a man?

No matter what our age or how our body looks, it is our self-esteem that will determine if we can let go of the self-deprecating thoughts long enough to have an orgasm when we do have someone lying beside us. Or, if we do, in fact, let someone lie next to us at all.

Look in the Mirror

Most books that discuss body image encourage you to quit looking in the mirror. I disagree. When I was at my heaviest, I did not own a full-length mirror . . . and I believe that contributed to my downward emotional spiral and my upward weight gain.

Mirrors are just mirrors. They are not here to judge us, but instead can give us the most accurate picture of our body that we are willing to see. What a gift that is! If we all lived in dimly lit rooms, flickering in candlelight, it would be easy to live in a fantasy. But fantasies have a way of blowing up in our faces, and in order to see what others see when we walk out the door into the sunlight, we must face what is happening to our bodies. We must know what we really look like in order to assess what we want to do in the future. For many of us, the mirror can be our first reality check.

Your Exercise

Learning to love yourself includes being willing to be with yourself exactly as you are, regardless of how you feel. So go ahead and look in the mirror right now. Do your best to leave your judgments behind. Start fully clothed if that is easier for you. But really look at your body. Your front, sides, back. Check out the curve of your hips, the strength of your torso, the power of your legs. Now grab a chair and sit down. I urge you to look at your body for a minimum of five minutes. Do not turn away.

If you are willing to be extra brave, strip down to your underwear. Look again. No one has your body. No one. No one has dimples in their cheeks exactly the same way that you do, whether it's on their face or on their butt. No one has the exact freckles. No one has the same scars because they have not had the same accidents, dents, and trips along the way.

Your body is the most visible form of uniqueness you possess. If you look closely, it is a road map of your life. The cellulite, the stiff shoulder, and the pain in your back are all yours. It's time to embrace them for being part of you. Because you can't truly let your body obsession go without being willing to love your body exactly as it is. That is a spiritual fact. We say we want to love ourselves, and many of us do tons of self-help work to feel loving toward ourselves, but now it's time to spread that love to include our bodies. I'm here to tell you that without an ability to love your body, including all your body parts, you will never love yourself. So, let's get to it. . . .

Sitting or standing in front of the mirror as naked as you possibly can get, just let your body know that you are willing to be on its side. And perhaps be willing to believe, maybe for the first time, it is on yours.

Sit or stand as long as you are able, and relish the opportunities your body gives you. What has your body taught you? How has your body changed over the years? What do you see now that wasn't there before? What pleasures have you experienced through your body that you couldn't experience otherwise? What gifts does your body share with you every day?

Mine has taught me patience, how to listen beyond words, and to pay attention. Three important skills that help me every day as the Life Coach in the *Starting Over* house. It has taught me to look beyond the surface, give up judgments, and love imperfections. Three skills I need to be happy.

This is the time to tell your body all the ways it has supported you. Be grateful. And if you find yourself getting angry before you can get grateful, honor that too. For the most part, our body only responds to what is placed upon it. Your body and mine are not the super bodies we had hoped for. In fact, they are more. They are miracle bodies, dodging our bad habits, repairing the damage we do, and loving us in spite of our behaviors.

When you are ready, I urge you to pick up a pen, grab a piece of paper, or jump on your computer and complete the following sentences.

I am most thankful for my body because ... *it lives, moves, sleeps, dances, gives birth, makes love ect..*

I am sorry I abused, hurt, or betrayed my body in the following ways ... *eating too much juck + not enough healthy stuff. Not erexcizings like I should,*

If I could hear my body tell me anything, I wish it would be ... *I am you - and I'm ready to experiance life - just do it!*

If I was willing to love my body, I would tell it ... *thanks - I'm lucky to have such health,*

As of late, I can say that I am doing all I can to be the best I can be physically, emotionally, mentally, and spiritually. Sometimes, it may be as little as putting down the fork when I am eating or getting off my tush when I am in the midst of feeling sorry for myself. Sometimes, it's replacing my negative body comments with gratitude or just looking at my body with love and telling it so. And let's not kid ourselves, there are still times that I must say "I'm sorry" for what I've said or done to hurt it in any way. The big difference between the past and the present is that I am truly learning to love myself, which adds compassion, tenderness, and kindness to my life. Qualities I need to be fearless.

I've gotten to the point where I like looking in the mirror again. I see my mother's body, and now, her face. I have her breasts, stomach, and even her smile. I am my mother. And I'm proud of that. She was beautiful, and so am I.

Oh, you might be wondering what happened to Ted. Well, nothing—yet. He has yet to ask me out. He still calls once in a while to ask how I am doing. As a matter of fact, he called last night. Both of us made small attempts at flirting, but no moves were made.

My "relationship," or lack thereof, with Ted, has awoken my

need, my desire, to share myself, including my body, with a man. I know now that I don't want my body to determine my capacity to love, but instead, I want my body to be able to express love, to share love. I think that's a good thing. So really, my distress about Ted really isn't about Ted. It's about not being enough, about being scared to fall in love, about growing old . . .

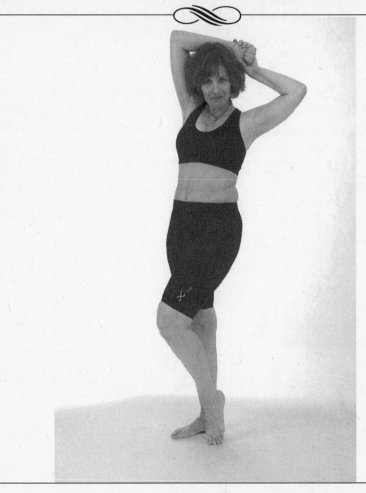

MARY ANN

Height: 5'9" • Weight: 165 pounds • Age: 54

Body Motto: *I want to work on making myself beautiful as I age from the inside out. I embrace the Goddess within me and the Goddess body I have right now.*

CHAPTER 7

How Do I Age Gracefully?

I wrote a book called *Fearless Living*.

I am all about being fearless.

I've built a career on helping people deal with their fears.

Nothing gives me more fulfillment.

Throughout the last twenty years, I've faced my greatest fears—and conquered many of them. Those that have lingered (primarily around issues with my body) you've been reading about in these pages.

But in writing this book, it became obvious that I couldn't talk about body image without dealing with one of the biggest fears that women of *all* body types share—aging. I've helped a lot of clients deal with this issue, so I can think of any number of stories to share with you. But it occurred to me that this chapter should be no different than the others—meaning, I'd have to talk about *myself*.

Until recently, I've never talked about my feelings on getting older. I've put aside my thoughts about what's happening and going to happen to my body, my health, and my energy. One thing is for certain: We're all getting older. So, let's be fearless here together and really look at what's ahead. . . .

If you're like me, there have been times in your life when you took your body for granted, thinking it would always do whatever you needed it to. I always figured that if I didn't think about it getting older, it somehow wouldn't happen. I wanted to believe that my body would do my bidding for the rest of my life with little worry or care. Skip across the railroad tracks? No problem. Run across the street super fast in order to avoid oncoming traffic? Can do. Stand on the kitchen counter to grab something off the top shelf? No danger there.

And then it happened. Reality hit me with a wake-up call. . . .

A lightbulb burnt out in the ceiling of my apartment. No biggie. I had changed plenty of lightbulbs in the past, so grabbing the nearest chair was of no concern. I just hopped on and stretched out my arms until the tips of my fingers just touched the screws holding the light fixture in place. I loosened one screw and then another. It was now at the critical juncture, the time to take out the third screw with my left hand while bracing the light fixture with my right. I carried on without even thinking about it.

And then I fell onto the linoleum. Hard. I couldn't believe it. Sprawled out on the kitchen floor, stuck in between the legs of the chair, I realized my body simply hadn't done as it was told. Thankfully I wasn't hurt. But I was shaken up. What the heck had happened?

After a day or two of walking around in a daze, I chalked it up to being too scattered, not paying enough attention to my surroundings. But this incident wasn't a fluke. Within a matter of weeks, it felt like I was inhabiting someone else's body. I'd walk down the street and trip for no reason. I fell getting out of the car one day in the rain, and missed a step going down some stairs. Overnight I had become a klutz—one of those people kids used to laugh at in school. Was I really just suddenly so unfocused that I couldn't walk a straight line without being in danger of spraining an ankle? No. Something else was going on. But *what*?

I went to the doctor for a physical, but he couldn't find a thing wrong with me. "You just fell," he said. "At your age, it's normal to trip from time to time, or miss a step." At *my* age?! I was only thirty-five years old. "Are you telling me that my body has already begun to betray me?" I didn't even wait to see if he had an answer for that before tuning him out by picking up a magazine and leafing through its pages. I was angry, and there was no way I was going to buy into the fact that it was all downhill from here.

On my drive home from that appointment, I realized that I had spent little time questioning what it took to have a balanced, physically fit body. I had expected to have control over myself for the rest of my life because of the simple fact that I had had it up until now. But apparently, age, years of neglect, and things like gravity have a cumulative effect. My body was slowly resisting being my obedient servant, and it was becoming obvious that I was going to have to change, or I could only expect more rebellion.

But just what was I supposed to do?

I started looking truthfully at the fact that, like many people, I had been the betrayer for years. Since the time I could remember, I had abused my body with unhealthy food choices, little exercise, and less than clean air. My mother didn't exercise, so being physical was not part of our family life. My father didn't fish or hike or run either, so I had no role models. I thought people just stayed young if they had good genes. And my family had good genes, or so I thought. My grandmothers both lived into their eighties, and my grandfathers passed away in their seventies. Somewhere in my brain, I thought I had received a get-out-of-jail-free card. But the jail was getting older—and so was I.

Role Models

As I often tell my clients, sometimes the best way to plan for the future is to look into the past. In looking back at mine, I can see why I've been avoiding this subject. As you know if you've read *Fearless Living* or heard any of my public speeches, my mother died a brutal death at the hands of my father when she was only thirty-nine years old. My father, who took his own life, died only minutes afterward, also at thirty-nine. Even though all teenagers think their parents are older than the hills, in reality, on the day of their deaths, my parents were still relatively young adults, and I was robbed of any firsthand experience of aging. I was left with no one to show me the ropes. Unable to see either of my parents go through the forties, fifties, sixties or beyond, my memories of them are basically frozen in time. A time when they were vibrant people—mostly on the younger side of the spectrum of life, still without lines, sagging skin, whitening hair, or any of the things we associate with age, like arthritis, dentures, baldness, age spots—you name it. I look back at pictures of my mom, and she was beautiful, healthy, and *thin*. She wore sleeveless shirts and had a pooch like I do, but she was one hot mama.

I identify more with my mother than my father for several reasons, but primarily in this instance because she, not he, was my gender role model. Mom will never age for me, and the weirdest concept is that even though she's still in her thirties in my mind (and always will be), I keep on aging, for the sheer fact that I'm alive! In my case, I am now officially older than my own mother.

I'll never forget the day I turned forty. That's a milestone for anybody, for sure, but for me, knowing that my mother died before her fortieth birthday made this a monumental day. I had grown up wondering, *Will I make it to forty?* The question was this thing—this weight—that hung over my head. When I got there, when I lived through the entire day, I was on top of the world. I was so grateful, so energized to have made it past the dreaded marker. And then it hit me: *I'm not sure how to do this . . . How does a woman live past forty? What does it look like to get older?*

Growing up, no one told me that starting off the morning with sugary cereal, soda, or a candy bar followed by junk food at every meal was a bad thing. I had no clue that sitting on the couch watching soap operas all day or reading for hours on end, without any physical exercise, could be hazardous to my health. It never occurred to me that if I didn't use my body, I could lose my body. Sure, I recognized unhealthy habits in other people, but somehow these examples never applied to *me.* I was in denial—especially when it came to cocktails in my roaring twenties. Didn't everyone drink to the extreme? Wasn't this the time of life to let loose and have fun? (Oh, the things an addictive personality will tell herself!) I thought my body was "Superbody," and thus, I could abuse it with little or no consequence. Because I hadn't seen anyone close to me age, I didn't think that getting older was going happen to me.

When I "fell from grace," as I began referring to my light bulb incident, my airy-fairy fantasy world crashed down with me. It was time to face reality—the reality of my body. And in the process, I realized a growing fear. If I couldn't trust my body to perform simple tasks on cue, what else was there in life that perhaps I couldn't trust?

No bones had been broken, for sure, but my ego and aspects of my self-confidence were sorely bruised. I felt far from invincible — vulnerable, even, and I was on the lookout for other problems in my life. If I could fall doing a simple household chore, couldn't another shoe drop, or slide out beneath me?

Expectations Become Reality

If you're like me, you have expectations of your body, how it should act, look, and age. Do you expect your legs to stay vein-free? What about arthritis, heart disease, cancer? Do you expect to be the lucky one to miss the family disease, or are you "destined" to get ill no matter what you do? Have you ever glanced at your family health history? And let's talk wrinkles. Do you curse your skin, or praise it? In my case, the expectations I had for my body were hidden from me until they were not met. Until I was disappointed in my body, and therefore myself, I didn't want to look. Now is the time for you to face the secret expectations you have been hoping would come true or dreading the inevitable but haven't been willing to take responsibility for. Expectations about our body, for most, are a source of heartache. Yet, no one seems to take claim for having them. Instead, they lie dormant, giving us ammunition to beat ourselves up for never being good enough.

Your Exercise

Please list the expectations you have for your body. How do you expect it to perform under stress? As you age? With various food choices and exercise plans? I have included a few starter sentences that might help trigger your brain into telling the truth. Above all, stay open and be thorough.

I expect my body to always . . .

I expect my body to never . . .

As I age, I expect my body to . . .

Based on my food choices, I expect my body to . . .

Based on my exercise regime, I expect my body to . . .

When I'm under stress, I expect my body to . . .

Because of my lifestyle choices, I expect my body to . . .

After reading this book and completing all the exercises, I expect my body to . . .

If you look at your list above, you may notice something that's subtle, but true for most of us. Our body and our sense of happiness are inextricably tied. The message I told myself after my fall was that my body was to blame for my latest insecurities and my inability to be happy. If I was having a "good body day," and everything looked great and acted accordingly, my happiness ensued. But the minute I glimpsed my mortality, through a mere trip or fall, I experienced fear and even anger. I didn't want to be that dependent. While I knew that I could not live without my body, I wasn't quite ready to admit that I was totally dependent on it, no matter how good it didn't look or how graceful it wasn't.

Your Family Aging Legacy

Many of our expectations are rooted in our family trees, including the hope of being wrinkle- and disease-free. Maybe you believe that expectations, facts, and genes are the same. Maybe you truly believe that your genes are a given and will produce certain events in your life no matter what you do. I imagine the sense of powerlessness you must feel and how that seeps into the rest of your life. Perhaps you think that if you can't control your body, how can you control any other aspect of your life, like your husband, kids, or your boss?

You might remember Allison from the *Starting Over* house. Before entering the house, she had her right breast removed due to cancer. She was scared of getting cancer again. Wait, that's not true. She *knew* she was going to relapse, and she just wanted to know how to handle it better. Her family tree was riddled with cancer and there was no way, in her mind, that she was going to escape the family "curse." Do you believe something similar? What is your fate, based on your family lineage? Cancer, like Allison? A heart attack by the age of what? Forty, fifty, sixty? Diabetes? Is that a given? Do you feel jinxed when family and friends tell you that you are "just like your mom"? Have you assumed that will mean you will die like her too?

Be honest. We all have our fears of getting old and some of those fears may connect to the way you might die. Because of the way my parents died, by my father's hand, I had a way out, an excuse for my denial (other than worrying that I might turn out crazy, like him). Are you like me, the person in denial who believes she can avoid any and all family patterns of aging? Whether you deny you will be like your mother, or just give into the inevitable, both take away your sense of personal freedom.

Over the years, I didn't know how to find the answers to my aging questions. Heck, I didn't even know who to go to for the normal questions—things like, "What do you do with bunions on your feet?" or "How do you tell the difference between a flu and a cold?" I was looking for the most basic information on aging and health, and was clueless.

I ended up learning about these things from my sisters and their friends. For instance, my sister Cindy taught me how to care for my face, including washing it first thing in the morning and last thing at night, how to apply moisturizer, and how important it is to wear sunscreen. Sometimes the questions my sisters and I discussed felt so embarrassing that we would whisper to each other while talking on the phone. I feel like I missed out on learning how to grow up and grow old. Half the time I still feel like I have no idea.

When I met my friend Marta, I was so relieved to have someone to go to who had this knowledge base. Someone whose mother had trained her well, and who could still ask her mother for guidance. I can't tell you how many times I called Marta and said, "What does this mean?" or "What do I do about that?" Even though I read every book I can get my hands on, I still look to Marta for answers. And I'm sure she has a chuckle once in a while about how "the big Life Coach" needs mothering. But what I've realized is that we all do.

While many of you reading this book still have mothers and female relatives to talk with, I'm sure a portion of you live a good distance from your mothers. These days, it's common to leave your hometown for school or work, and to see your parents mostly on special occasion. Some of you aren't sure where your mother is, or like me, your mother passed away before you had a chance to ask. If you're not witnessing the aging process up close and personal, it's easier to deny, and therefore it's easier to get caught by surprise when your denial no longer works.

To gain that knowledge, I recommend that my clients who aren't in close physical proximity to their mothers (and now, possibly you) find a mentor—a friend or relative who can lead the way. If that's not possible, reading about the subject does wonders for opening up the mind. Age, I'm finding, isn't so scary when you understand it. Knowledge can erase much of our fear.

One thing I have learned through all my the research is how much power we have over our body. Our food choices, exercise plan, ability to manage stress, nutritional support, and the environment around us make a huge impact on whether our family cancer gene manifests or not. These factors also affect our aging process. The way we care for the inside of our bodies will help determine how our outsides look and how we feel about our body as a whole.

"You Look Great for Your Age!"

As you might have guessed, so many of the things we've talked about in this book—habits for feeling thinner, healthier, and more energetic—are the very things that will help you age more gracefully. But don't be surprised if people can't quite register your healthy habits with your climbing age. A client of mine, Diane, has a beautiful daughter and a handsome husband. She used to be an actress and modeled a bit on the side. Her friends consider her a lucky woman, "good genes" they say, but it's easy to see that Diane did not "luck into" her life and her looks. She has worked for them day in and day out. In taking good care of her body by eating well, carrying out work she loves, getting plenty of rest, and finding the time to squeeze a workout into her hectic life, Diane has done as good a job as anyone at stalling the inevitable. People say to her, "You look so great for fifty-two!" as if it's a miracle that fifty-two looks great. People say that to me sometimes: "You look amazing for forty-five!" I want to say, "Why can't I just look great? Why do looks have to be in relation to age?"

The media barrage us with ads all day long that tell us how to look younger, with the underlying message that being younger is better. As women, we are told to lie about our age, otherwise we could be kicked out of our careers before we're ready. Like an earthquake that could strike any time, we never know when our time is up.

How are we supposed to be proud of who we are, yet be okay with lying about our age? The hypocrisy in this thinking hits at the very core of who I am. It doesn't make sense. It doesn't seem right. It smacks of lack of integrity. I refuse to lie. For the record, I am forty-five years old and my birthday is December 1. There, that's done. Will you follow suit?

What exactly is forty-five supposed to look like, anyway? It's as if we all still think that being "old" means being hunched over a cane, with white hair, and wearing itty-bitty glasses—like my grandma. Even though sixty is the new fifty, and fifty is the new forty, and so on . . . that's not the point. Why can't we claim our older years, love our bodies, and be happy no matter what? It's time to create new images!

I'm all for staying healthy, living as long as possible, and looking my best. Yes, I do want to feel young, but not at the expense of my worth, my value, my self-esteem. Sadly, this isn't the case for everyone. Ask yourself, do you hide your age or are you proud of it? When you receive a compliment, do you mumble something about how old you look and complain about the cottage cheese on your thighs, or do you smile and say thank you . . . and mean it?

Working together is the only way we will shift the world's view on aging. As women, we have an obligation to the women who have gone before us and the women who will follow, to honor our bodies and break the legacy of self-hatred and disgrace that we place upon our bodies daily. If we are ever going to reach our potential as women, we must begin to heal the bodies we use to move around in this world. They are part of us, a gift to us, and something that is meant to be used with pride rather than disdain. But that is up to us. Each of us must be willing to let go of the shame that gives us permission to betray ourselves and one another. As we age, we need to join forces and come closer to each other rather than farther apart. We must celebrate all of who we are and all our glory, otherwise we are giving less than we could to the healing of the planet.

With ad campaigns reaching the billions and covers of mainstream women's magazines focused on beauty and fashion rather than personality and achievements, we are in trouble. Today I was glancing through the latest edition of one of my favorite women's magazines aimed at, or so I thought, women of substance. Inside they had a fascinating article on a fascinating woman, someone I admire and respect for her contributions to business, creativity, and being a woman who holds her own with men. I enjoyed the article thoroughly. Did this amazing woman make the cover? Nope. Was she even a secondary headline? Nope. Instead, the story was tucked in between the hottest beauty dos and don'ts, and the latest health craze. What *was* on the cover? The winner of their latest model search. I wanted to cry. It's no wonder that, as women, our body image and age are on our minds twenty-four hours a day, seven days a week. The message we receive: If you want to be seen in this world, it won't be through your mind or heart; it will be through your looks.

Your Real Age

Okay, so let's have it. What is your chronological age versus your biological age versus how old you feel?

For me, those are all very different ages. My chronological age is forty-five, but my biological age is somewhere in my mid-thirties due to my now healthy lifestyle: eating five servings of veggies a day, lifting weights regularly, moving my body daily, staying positive, and letting go of stress. But mentally, I feel nineteen years old half the time. To be perfectly frank, I do not want to look, feel, or act "old," and sometimes that can get me into trouble. I can be guilty of dressing younger than my age in the quest to appear more youthful. I have been known to walk into the juniors department with my nineteen-year-old nieces, Rachel and Deena, and actually plop down money to get the same thing they do. I am forty-five years old. I know I shouldn't, and they let me know it's wrong by their look of shock (mixed with a little disgust along with a giggle or two). But I can't help myself; I forget I'm forty-five because inside, I still feel nineteen.

When I am hanging around with my nieces, I almost forget the age differences between us. Okay, I *want* to forget the age differences and just be one of the girls. I want to forget that my body isn't the same as it once was. In reality, it usually becomes abundantly clear to me the minute I bring that junior item into the dressing room and check myself out in the three-way mirror. Instead of feeling good, it just makes me feel old. And that is exactly what I don't want to feel.

Truth be told, I don't think aging would be so bad if my body didn't have to get old. When I lie in bed at night, I sometimes imagine that I have the body of my youth. It's easier to have this fantasy lying down than when I'm walking around upright. When I'm lying down, all of my excess weight melts into the mattress (along with my less-than-wonderful body confidence). I can't feel my thighs rubbing together or the weight of gravity on my back, and I feel weightless. But I know the truth will return in the morning when the lights go up, and that's when I know I must pray for health, wisdom, and love. Those are the things I really want—even more than a young, tight body. I just wish I could be that enlightened during the daytime, when all the lights are on.

It would be nice to say that my fear of aging has stopped completely. If only life were that simple. But my fears of getting older and "less than" haven't stopped because I've become successful. They haven't stopped because I use the most advanced anti-aging products. It's ironic. After my parents died, I spent ten years trying to figure out how to kill myself. I wanted nothing more than to die an early death and be reunited with my beautiful mother. But now that I've learned how to live a mostly fearless life, I want to relish life. There's so much I want to experience, to give, to accomplish. Aging is a fact of life that I'm doing my best to face, and I will not let it stop me from being fully myself.

Truth be told, I am no longer afraid to die. It feels good to say it out loud. Kind of scary, too. I realized years ago that I do not want to be so afraid to die that I forget to live. So to stay focused on living, I write down my obituary every year. It tells me quickly what matters in my life and reminds me to live and age with grace, ease, and a commitment to what matters most. Sure, it's part fantasy and part reality, but it gives me focus and hope, reminds me what I hope the world sees when they see me. (Notice that no obituary mentions the wrinkles on our skin or our weight. I guess that doesn't matter when we are dead, why does it matter when we are alive?)

Think about it. What do you want your last words to be? What legacy do you want to leave your family and friends? How do you want to be remembered?

My Latest Obituary:

Rhonda Britten, age 110, died today from natural causes. According to friends and family, she passed away in her sleep after a day of hiking with her nieces, a day filled with laughter, love, and family. Her second husband told reporters: "This is exactly how Rhonda would have wanted to die. I'd like to thank her fans for their notes, flowers, and cards. It means so much to the family that she had such an effect on the world. She will be remembered and sorely missed."

Britten was one of the most popular talk-show hosts of this century and still considered one of the most influential women on the globe. The president of the United States declared the day of her death "Fearless Day" to commemorate all of her tireless work in the area of fear, requesting that the nation lower its flags to half-staff.

Her favorite accomplishments included being named *Time* magazine's Woman of the Year, being appointed to the President's Council on Women's Issues, being UN Special Representative for Fearless Technologies (influencing the way the world communicates), and continuing to make a difference worldwide as the founder of the Fearless Living Institute.

But to Rhonda, her greatest accomplishment was the healing of her family legacy and her commitment to change the way women see themselves in the world.

Her funeral will be held at her family home. Attending will be her second husband with their three children, seven grandchildren, and thirteen great-grandchildren, along with her two sisters, their husbands and children, Rhonda's nieces and nephews, Jason, Rachel, Deena, Adam, and Zachary, along with their families. Her ashes will be scattered in Lake Superior at the height of fall amongst the fall leaves.

Sigh! I always well up when I am writing my obituary because I'm writing from my heart about my future, about what I want my life to be about. It gives me goals and forces me to think big. And yes, I'm mixing a little fantasy in, but who knows, maybe it could happen!

Somehow, between children and menopause, we are supposed to stay young, stay firm, and stay wrinkle-free. I feel sandwiched in between the expectations of society and the reality of growing older. Add to that my own body insecurities and you have a recipe for low body confidence, lower self-esteem, and in some strange way, the pathway to self-love—which I will discuss in an upcoming chapter.

My body will age, it's a biological foregone conclusion. But it doesn't mean I have to feel old or despise my body along the way. You have a lot of power over your body even when it comes to the rate at which you age. And it will be up to you to decide how aging will affect you. I know I've decided to embrace my age, relish my wisdom, and honor my youth. I know that's what my parents would wish for me, and that's what I wish for my nieces, and now, for you. . . .

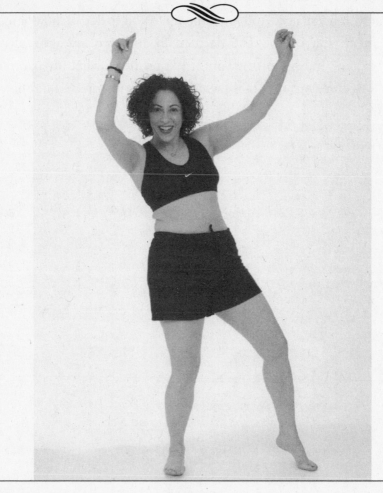

JODI

Height: 5'5" • Weight: 157 pounds • Age: 46

Body Thoughts: *I'm grateful for my state of mind about my body. As I get healthier, I appreciate what I have and who I am now. I'm not so concerned about every little bump and bulge anymore.*

CHAPTER 8

How Can I Take Responsibility for My Body?

I've been thinking about how, as a nation, we Americans seem to talk about religion and spirituality nonstop, and tout our values on big ol' neon signs. But for all the increased consciousness and evolved souls this nation is supposed to contain, why don't our bodies match our spirits?

As I've shared before, we have more obesity than ever before, and for that matter, more anorexia, bulimia, and various other eating disorders. It's like God granted us the land of plenty, and we don't know how to handle it. We are on sensory overload—or should I say, food overload. We are out of control emotionally and physically while trying to keep it all together spiritually. Something isn't right.

I think the world needs more love. Pure and simple. Love of each other. Love of ourselves. We need to know we are loved. We all know, intellectually, that we have to love ourselves first before we will ever truly feel loved by another. The problem is that we don't allow ourselves to have it, to let it in. Somewhere inside of us we don't think we deserve it.

Most people would agree that the number one quality they want in a mate is a great sense of humor. Yet, we reject people because of the color of their hair, the clothes on their backs, or the shoes on their feet. We don't like the way they sniffle or how they open the car door, if they open the car door. We talk about the qualities we seek in a person, but when it comes down to taking the time to get to know someone, we balk. And that includes ourselves. It just feels too scary. We don't know what to do, so we end up eating. Pass the french fries, please!

We've all had the experience when we've gotten to know people who had such great personalities that, after a few twirls around the dance floor, they became more attractive to us, and we started seeing them as a potential partner. All of a sudden we couldn't care less about their looks, their weight, or their checkbook. (We've also all known gorgeous people who become ugly to us through their words and deeds.) But in most cases, we have a tough time getting beyond the surface when it comes to opening ourselves up to love. We hope that what's inside of us matters as much, if not more, than our exterior, but we devalue the importance of our own character (and obsess about things that are out of our control).

Isn't that what we complain about? We complain that men are shallow. That our boss doesn't appreciate us. That our children take us for granted. Now, replace the words "men," "boss," and "children" with the word "you." You are shallow. You don't appreciate you. You take you for granted.

As women, we don't give ourselves credit for our accomplishments, regardless of our size. We don't look at ourselves in amazement. We aren't thankful for who we are, regardless of our past. We don't make our dreams come true, no matter what our bodies look like. Rather, we scorn, hurt, and generally punish ourselves for not being more perfect.

We obsess about our looks, but get mad when others do the same. We want someone to see our heart, but we cover it up with clothes that don't fit and hair that is beyond any recognition of natural. We don't take care of ourselves the best we can, yet wonder when someone will come along and do just that. We want others to go first, to make us *feel* worthy, but that's not the way it works. Instead, we have to know our own worth because then we will have the type of worthiness that no one will ever be able to take away from us.

I understand it is hard, especially when you feel so stuck, so out of shape, so worthless. It doesn't help that we live in a visual society. We watch TV, we attend movies, we read magazines. We're visual. Men are extremely visual. Here we are in a visual society, saying that looks shouldn't matter. What's a person to do?

We *are* our body, all of it. And yes, we are more than our bodies. It's time for you to take responsibility for what you've done (and haven't done) for your body, and to your body. It's time to take your body back.

In the previous chapters, we've talked about the nation's health, or lack thereof. We've discussed belief systems, excuses, and even sex. Now it's time to address our own unwillingness to take responsibility for our lives. Your body is a part of your life, a big part. Like I've said, it determines so much of who we have become. So how can we start to take responsibility for our bodies?

What Part of You Is Your Body Expressing?

Our bodies are a barometer, a manifestation of how we feel about ourselves. If you think your arms are fat, you're probably holding them back, not reaching out or embracing people or things. If you think your thighs are elephant huge, can you really swing your hips with the best of them? (For your information, hips are meant to swing!)

Think about how safe you feel in the world. Many times we use our bodies to protect us when we don't know any other way to do it. Little girls who have been abused can become adults who feel compelled to stay safe with a layer of protection called fat. Or perhaps you have a difficult time saying no or feel uncomfortable with conflict? You might be like Allison in the *Starting Over* house, who gained weight, unconsciously of course, to make sure no one would want to date her. Allison didn't trust herself when it came to men, so this became an easy excuse that just rolled off her tongue: "Oh no, I don't date. Look at me." Maybe you are like me and gained weight to blame yourself for your loveless marriage.

On the other hand, it's important to remember the ways your body supports you, regardless of your opinions about its appearance. When we feel love, we use our body to hug, kiss, and speak kind words to our loved ones. If we are giddy, our feet skip, glide, and dance, allowing us to express our joy. Unresolved grief may cause our body to be tired because of the unexpressed emotion we are suppressing, while anger may make our body tight like a drum. The body manifests our emotions, and our emotions, when denied, manifest within our body. Our outer body and our inner life create our existence.

So many of us gain weight, lose weight, hold on to weight, abuse our weight, deny our weight, ignore our weight—all under the pretense of being too busy, too important, too poor, too spiritually evolved to deal with such a human problem.

My motto: The more I embrace my humanity, the more I experience the divine. And that includes my relationship with my body.

When I embrace my humanity, I am free to experience my feelings and face my fears. I must be willing to look at my body as an expression of who I am. Just like an artist, you and I have been given a body that has been our very first canvas. We can paint it (with makeup), draw on it (with tattoos), dress it up or dress it down (with clothes), primp it up (with handbags, four-inch heels, and combs with bling), and top it off with something that makes us feel sexy, serious, or whatever we decide (dreadlocks, blonde highlights, red streaks).

As you glance at yourself in the mirror, ask yourself what part of your personality you are expressing. The self-deprecating part, the creative essence, the business maven, or something else?

Your Exercise

I challenge you, urge you, invite you to focus on what you *do* have going for you. Focus on your intelligence. Focus on your humor. What do you like about you? What do people say that they love about you? Take a few minutes and list the top ten compliments you have received lately or the good things you hope you have (but might be afraid to admit). I'm not asking you to agree with them. That will take time. But I am asking you to acknowledge them and, just for now, contemplate the fact that they *might* be true. Some of mine are: People compliment me on my eyes. I've been told I have heart when I am working on a project. I have good handwriting. I can stand on one leg a really long time.

1.
2.
3.
4.
5.
6.
7.
8.
9.
10.

Good, now we are heading in the right direction!

The Path of Self-Hatred

Now we're approaching the crux of this work. I have had clients come to my office and swear they like themselves. It's just their body they hate. Does that make any sense to you? Or maybe it rings a bell with you? It just might be one of the craziest lines of thinking any of us get into!

Let's go back to Bethany in the *Starting Over* house—remember the "big boned" young woman who had lost her memory? As she faced her inner demons, she could no longer hide from her body hatred even though, believe me, she tried! Until that pivotal moment, Bethany had denied having an issue with her body. Sure, she had said that she wanted to lose weight. And yes, she didn't like the scar on her belly from her surgery, just like me. But hate her body? Bethany was way too kind and good-hearted to admit such a horrible truth.

But she did admit she hated herself. I mentioned that might include her body. She nodded in silent agreement. It was time for Bethany to take responsibility for the things she said and did, as well as all the excuses in between.

At the *Starting Over* house I sometimes have to get creative to make a point and today was one of those days. I led Bethany to a thick plaster faux-brick wall I had built in order to show her what she had been doing to herself. She had been blocking her own growth, and I wanted that brick wall to block our path as we strolled outside the *Starting Over* house. It was the perfect metaphor for Bethany's life. "That's exactly how I feel," she said in her Southern accent. "I feel like there is an invisible brick wall between me and my future and I can't figure out why it keeps getting in my way." I could hear the frustration in her voice.

"I'm glad you are willing to admit that," I said. "Now, are you willing to admit the things you tell yourself about yourself? I dare you to write down all the words and phrases that enter your head when you want to take a risk. Go on." And with that I handed her a can of spray paint, and she began to graffiti the wall with her disempowering statements.

You know you hate your body when you call yourself, as Bethany did that day, "ugly," "stupid," and "disgusting." Bethany also compared herself to her younger sister, Jessica. Jessica was a petite, dark-hair beauty who went to college right out of high school. Bethany felt like a loser being four years older than her baby sis and still afraid to go to college. This had become so engrained into her psyche that she believed she deserved to be behind Jessica in everything from school to boys. In other words, Bethany didn't believe she was good enough.

In big fluorescent-orange letters Bethany wrote across the wall, "I hate myself." It had come to that, as it does for many of us if we are honest. Since she woke up with amnesia, Bethany had daily headaches that could quickly turn into migraines, and she had a stomachache all the time. Sure, she'd been to the doctors, but nothing gave her immediate relief. By the time I met Bethany, she had given up on doing anything about it. She figured she'd have to live the rest of her life with an upset stomach and a throbbing head. Somehow that was fine with her. It was not fine with me.

Bethany is the perfect example of someone who put up with ill health because she was tired of dealing with it. In her mind, she wasn't *worth* the effort. She hated herself for being stuck in a body that she feared was never going to get well, and in some ways feared that she had created.

Self-hatred had stopped her cold and given her permission to call herself the worst of names. I knew that if she didn't discover the path of self-love soon, Bethany would never make it to college, find love, or look in the mirror with anything but disdain.

To discover what self-hatred looked like, I asked her to take another stroll with me through Griffith Park, the largest green belt inside the Los Angeles city limits. As we made our way under towering trees alongside a babbling creek, we came upon a sign that read CHOICE.

The sign pointed to two pathways: SELF-HATRED and SELF-LOVE.

Of course Bethany immediately wanted to choose SELF-LOVE, but I cautioned her. I told her that there are things you must commit to if you walk that path, and that first, it was time she understood the path she was familiar with: SELF-HATRED.

The SELF-HATRED path led us across a river, up a hill, and across some difficult terrain. "Is this how it feels to live your life?" I asked. "Are you always jumping over obstacles, feeling like life is an uphill battle and everything is hard?" She nodded. I could tell there was someplace inside of her that wanted to keep blaming her body for her failed plans. Instead, I wanted her to face how her self-hatred might be the reason for her misery.

We came upon our first marker on the Path of Self-Hatred: ISO-LATES SELF. Bethany could not argue with that. When she lost her memory, she gave up on college and left any friends from the past in the dust. She was too embarrassed to be friends with anyone. She had no support team, no confidantes, no anybody. She felt like a burden. Bethany had become an expert at being alone.

As we walked on, the next marker rose up from the shrubbery reading: PRETENDS TO BE HAPPY. Another sign of Self-Hatred. Bethany had a void all right—her memory. But that wasn't all. She had created other voids in her life—voids like dating and just plain fun, things every young girl should experience. She compensated by filling her voids with food, negative self-talk, and work that was "just a job," not a career she was passionate about.

Marker number three was simple to understand: MAKES EX-CUSES. Bethany had plenty of those. She had decided she wasn't smart enough for college, even though she had received a college scholarship and was a straight-A student before her amnesia. She thought everyone was being nice to her because they felt sorry for her, even though before her illness she had tons of friends who cared and a church full of people who knew her name. Also she believed she was the ugliest creature on earth, even though just a few days before her amnesia struck she had been crowned the local county beauty queen. She felt nothing was right, especially not Bethany.

As we walked on, marker number four could be seen in the distance, surrounded by a garden of wildflowers. SETTLES was the last and final sign showing that she was on the Path of Self-Hatred. Bethany began to weep. "I get it, Rhonda. I've been so unhappy and I didn't want to admit it." She finally understood that in her own way, she had been making unhappiness her goal. Her excuses, her void, her isolation, and her desire to settle were all ways she kept herself miserable. It was her self-hatred that was keeping her stuck, not her amnesia or her headaches or her body.

Are You on the Same Path?

Are you following the same markers that Bethany did? Is your misery a badge of honor that proves you don't deserve happiness?

I remember the words I said to my then-husband when I realized what I was asking Bethany to realize now: "I am no longer willing to be unhappy to get your love." I hope the same becomes true for you. Your happiness is not for sale. Ever. It is your birthright to be madly, passionately, ecstatically happy with no regrets, no excuses. Nobody's love is worth that much.

Just like with Bethany, your body and how you feel about it guides every decision you make. So take responsibility for it and choose to love it. You are your body, whether you like it or not: The mirror does not lie. *Your* body is staring back at you, not the airbrushed image you might have in your head, an image that will "show up" the moment you give up sugar, get more sleep, or lose that weight. This is good news, because as soon as you get real and take responsibility for your body as is, it can finally take responsibility for you.

However, it needs your help. *Help your body to help you!* With better, more loving decisions, it can help you stay around a lot longer, and you'll both be happier throughout the journey.

I'd like you to stop for a minute and think about what you just read. *You* are responsible for your body. Don't give me that "Yeah, yeah, yeah" reaction. I did that brush-off myself for years, complete with eye rolling. However, that arrogant denial still catches up with me because there is no abusing our bodies without consequences.

I understand you've had help. Maybe you gave up taking care of yourself like you used to after your third baby because you were just too tired. Perhaps it happened after you were fired from your job because you didn't feel like you could afford or were worth any self-care. You could, in your mind, be trying hard right now and have no idea what I'm talking about. Maybe you're thinking: "I *do* take responsibility for my body." Well, super. I hope that's true. But are you sure you are taking responsibility for your body, or do you *think* you are taking responsibility because you are hard on yourself? That is not responsibility. And it's definitely not loving.

In case you're still trying to get around this one, I'm going to say it one last time: YOU ARE RESPONSIBLE FOR YOUR BODY. Some of you will want your body to be responsible for *you*, and in many ways it is. But it's not a magician, and it can only hold danger at bay for so long. Just like a dam built to hold water back from flooding the plains, it can only do what it was made to do. Once the damage becomes too great, the water overflows . . . and we get sick.

Some people get mad when their body fights back or breaks down. Some want to get even by treating it more harshly, just like Bethany did. Poor food choices, soda after soda all day long, little sleep, and stress to the hilt will catch up with you. I want you to think about your last week. How many times in the last seven days were you mad at your body? Be honest with yourself. Do you remember looking in the mirror and shaking your head? At any time did you wish your stomach or thighs or arms were different? Did you call your body a name? Blame it for making you miserable? Curse it for being less than someone else's body?

Really think about this. How many times did you apologize for having your body to others, calling it fat, lazy, smelly, pale, swollen, ugly, unkempt? How many times did you hide it from friends or your spouse or yourself? How many times did you brush off compliments? How many times did you abuse it with too much food, alcohol, drugs—or not enough nutritious food or medicine? If you can't count that high, rest assured you are not alone.

What if you are of the belief that *"You are not your body; you are more than your body."* Let's take the phrase "You are more than your body" and break it down. What does it really mean? Regardless of your spiritual upbringing or your religious beliefs, I think we can all agree that our body can be viewed as a vehicle to do our higher purpose, our divine work here on earth. Without physical form, we cannot fulfill our purpose, our destiny, or our passion.

Does that mean that we are only capable of doing good in the world if we have a strong, healthy body? Of course not. Thankfully, we do not have to be limited by the capacities of just our physical bodies. Think of Christopher Reeve. After he became paralyzed, in some ways, he did his most important work. He became more in tune to life, more passionate, more determined than when his body was completely healthy. There are so many examples of extraordinary people who have limited use of their bodies, but they do have a body, *their* body. And trust me, anyone who can get beyond physical limitations and lead a happy, productive life is a role model for all of us. The folks who deal with chronic pain, a broken back or, like Bethany, daily headaches, are inspiring. When we don't use our bodies fully and completely, loving them with all our heart, it's as if, dare I say it, we're telling God, "Thank you, but no thank you. I'd like a different model, please, and when I get it, then I will fulfill my purpose, fall in love, and grow a garden."

That is how I felt. Until I decided to make another choice. You have the opportunity now. It's time to commit to being a loving partner to your body. It's time to commit to taking an action that could change your life. It's time to learn to listen to your body.

Listen to Your Body

Our body is our greatest ally in facing the world around us. If we listen to it and take care of its needs, it will take good care of us in return by giving us the opportunity for a healthier, longer, more satisfying life.

"What do you mean, listen to it?" my client Jessica asked. She had never heard of the concept of "listening to your body."

"It's talking to you all the time," I said, "but you're probably refusing to listen. Most of us don't want to face the changes our bodies are asking us to make." She didn't seem to be following a word of what I was saying, but I hadn't either when I was in her place.

In the third *Starting Over* house, Jessica wanted to heal from the death of her mother, which was especially hard because her mother hadn't died of natural causes or a long illness. Her dear, sweet, fifty-two-year-old mom died in the tragedy of 9/11. She was flying from Boston to San Francisco to take care of her elderly mother and had no idea when she boarded her flight that it would be the first plane to hit tower one of the World Trade Center. Jessica believed that she had dealt with her mother's passing but her body kept giving her a different message: anxiety. Within the first few minutes of meeting her, it was obvious that Jessica was jumpy and nervous—filled with fear.

I told Jessica that our bodies are to be trusted. They are the true barometer of our emotional life. She thought she was fine, but her body didn't agree. In the past, when Jessica became anxious, she would freeze up or give up. I showed her that by listening to her body, she could actually move through her feelings rather than deny them, her giving the courage to get past them rather than use them as an excuse. I believe in the theory that *in order to get over it, you have to go through it*, and that includes your body.

I want you to start listening to your body. If you can, look at it with as little judgment as possible. It will begin to talk to you. If you really pay attention, it will begin sharing with you its pains, heartaches, and disappointments. And it will also begin telling you what it wants. What it needs.

We're afraid to feel our disappointment and our past hurts because they remind us of times gone by. Your sagging breasts and wide hips may remind you of how heartbroken you were when your husband left you for a younger woman after you had two kids. Looking at your fat thighs may remind you that you are just like your mother and she talked down to you as a kid. Your big booty may be a visual reminder of how the boys teased you for being the chubby one in school. Or maybe the boys loved you for your athletic, firm butt—the one that no longer lives anywhere but in your memories. There are a million and one things our bodies remind us of, and that's why it feels so easy to emotionally beat your body up, put it down, and generally abuse it. The alternative would be to feel what you are deathly afraid of. Yet, that is the only way to freedom.

So go ahead: look and listen. What is your body trying to tell you? What is the cellulite on your skin telling you it needs or wants? What about the laugh lines around your eyes? Can you give your legs some credit for helping you walk farther than your mind wants to at times?

The Risk of Career Change

As my marriage began to fall apart, and having a baby seemed like a Band-Aid that wouldn't stick anyway, I realized there was something brewing inside of me fueling my need to overeat. I had begun coaching clients just months before, and I was in the process of planning workshops. But I had a dilemma. My husband didn't want me, so how could I expect the public to want to get coaching from a loser? (Or should I say, a gainer who was getting dumped?)

I worried. *What can I teach anyone, anyway? Look at my life! My husband is walking out the door. I am so out of shape, how can I hold workshops in my house? Great,* I thought to myself. *This is fantastic. Gaining weight has ruined every aspect of my life.*

I imagined potential clients laughing behind my back, whispering:

"Who would want her life? Why should we listen to her?"

"Her husband doesn't even want her!"

"Well, you can see why. She's too heavy to be enlightened."

"Who does she think she is, trying to coach? Rhonda's the one who needs a coach!"

I tried to fight back. *Okay, so I'm heavy,* I admitted to myself.

But people have told me that I give great advice and that they want to learn from me. I need to remember my motto: "Accept their words at face value," which means accept a compliment as true, and do not add your own interpretation. Right then, that was hard to imagine.

Being ashamed of who we are seduces us into believing that if we were better, thinner, or just more of *something*, life would work out for us. So we opt for a lifestyle rather than a life. We go for the material possessions of success instead of courting what matters more: a healthy sense of self.

I had to ask myself, what was it that was standing between me and my dream of building a thriving coaching practice? The answer came through loud and clear: my dang body.

Take Back Your Body

I knew then that I had to take my body back. I figured that if I wanted to save my marriage and have a career, my body was the key. I had to quit using it as the reason my life was stalled. I could change the way I ate—*if I wanted to*. I could get off the couch and exercise—*if I wanted to*. I could decide to be open, vulnerable, and honest—*if I wanted to*.

It was up to me, *and I wanted to*.

I remember getting off the scale for the umpteenth time after seeing no positive change, and walking to the refrigerator, overwhelmed with a feeling of doom. *I have no will power. I have no discipline. I don't deserve happiness. I can't lose weight. My body is the enemy.* I sat on the floor and started to cry. I felt so powerless sprawled out on the floor. I started to ask myself once again why I couldn't figure this out. What was so wrong with me that I couldn't keep my life together?

I know that the greatest lessons of our life are the lessons we don't want to learn. *Perhaps this is one of them,* I thought. *Perhaps I am supposed to learn something from my weight.* With nothing to lose, I grabbed a piece of paper and wrote down the following question:

God, what is the purpose of this weight?

Much to my surprise, an answer came. I could hear it plain and clear.

"My child," the voice said. I was sure it was God. "Without the weight, you wouldn't realize how smart you are, how wanted you are, or how magnificent you are. Your worth is not tied to your weight. But you don't know that yet. You had to gain weight in order to begin to truly love yourself."

I was dumbfounded. "What do you mean, 'realize how wanted I am'? My husband doesn't want me." This made no sense. I kept asking, and the answers kept coming.

"Rhonda," the voice continued, "you have used your body to get what you want all your life. To get a man. To get a career. But now that it has changed, you don't want it. If only you were thin, you tell yourself, then your life would work. But being thin isn't the answer, because your body isn't the problem. *You* are. You don't believe you are enough exactly as you are. You don't believe you are smart unless you are thin. You don't believe people will come to you or that your husband loves you unless you are thin. There is no weight standing in your way. Your weight is here to help you realize that you have everything you need already. Are you listening?"

With tears streaming down my cheeks, I realized that God was right. When I was younger, I had always used my body to get what I wanted. I thought it was my only asset, and without it, I had no way to make my dreams come true. My body meant power. And with my added pounds, I felt powerless. I started to see that maybe that wasn't the case at all.

At that moment, I decided to quit blaming my body for my problems and instead face my fear of not being enough. I was good enough, exactly as I was. I made my first flyer that evening for a workshop that I would have in my home a month from that day. I quit watching every move my husband made toward me (or didn't make, rather), and I made the move. I went over to my husband and kissed him, hard. Expecting nothing in return.

I would like to say that he responded warmly and in kind. I would love to say we lived happily ever after. We didn't, of course. But I did. The shame of my weight was released when I could look at my body and honestly say, thank you. Thank you for loving me enough to teach me that I am enough, exactly as I am.

Your Body Is a Teacher

Learning to look at your body as a teacher is an important step. Every pound we curse is connected to the shame we feel about who we are. I asked Summer, a *Starting Over* housemate, to face her shame with a wheelbarrow and a shovel.

There's nothing pretty about a mound of fat staring at you from the bottom of a wheelbarrow, but that was what Summer was facing on a hot autumn day at the *Starting Over* house. She kept telling me session after session that she didn't know why she gained weight; at one point, she even had a difficult time admitting that she had food issues, even though she would gobble down chips after her workouts or forget about drinking water altogether. Her refusal to complete her food diary told me she was hiding something, she was abusing her body. But today was going to be different. I wanted her to speak from her heart and tell me, pound by pound, what her weight meant to her. What it represented.

Summer looked like she was going to throw up when I asked her to grab the shovel and start emptying the fifty-pound glob inside the wheelbarrow. As I pointed to the lard that represented her excess weight, I asked her to share the real reason she had gained the weight. It was for a reason. And most likely for a good reason.

At first, it was difficult for Summer to admit that her excess weight represented anything at all. Who wants to admit that you've gained weight because your boyfriend dumped you or you were laughed at in gym class? I understood her hesitation, but I wasn't Summer's friend, I was her Life Coach, and it was time for Summer to take responsibility for her continuing abuse toward her body, toward her soul, toward herself.

With wild abandon, she starting flinging the lard from the wheelbarrow onto the tarp I had laid on the grass for this specific purpose. Pound after pound, she declared aloud how every pound was attached to a pain, a hurt, a shameful memory. She named them one by one, each event, each experience, as if it were happening now. She got angry. Really angry.

Most people don't want to deal with their own anger, let alone anyone else's. But we all need to feel our anger when it comes up, instead of running away. Think of it this way: Anger is just power. Power that you are choosing to channel as anger because you feel powerless, frustrated, and you want things to change. But maybe you don't know how to change things, so you get angry. Anger, in and of itself, isn't bad. What's bad is our inability to channel it for our good.

When Summer was getting mad, I kept telling her to go with it, to get angry, but to use that energy to slap that lard onto the tarp and tell it exactly what she thought. Summer had been turning the anger inward, giving her the motivation to grab another cupcake or bag of chips when what she really wanted was a hug, a touch, understanding.

Summer isn't the only one. When we are hurt or angry, most of us refuse to express it because we are petrified of the power behind it. We don't know what to do, so we stuff it, literally, in our thighs, our hips, our hearts.

Summer, like so many of us, had gained weight to avoid rejection. She gained weight to deny her pain. She put the pounds on when she was felt, confused, and scared. Just like me, Summer wanted to do the healthy thing, the right thing, but she didn't know how, and her real needs, felt too overwhelming to change.

It was now time to learn the lessons meant for her.

I asked Summer to review the benefits of gaining weight and to find the lesson she might learn from it all. There's always a benefit in everything we do, even if it appears to be a negative, like weight gain or negative self-talk. For Summer, it was difficult at first to find a lesson inside her extra fifty-plus pounds, but she persevered. What did her weight teach her? That her heart was tender and she was afraid of it being broken. Her weight was her protection from getting too dizzy-headed or feeling out of control when it came to love. Her extra pounds kept her focused on things not people. Her career kept her ambitious and motivated to learn everything she could about how to make money and be successful. In some ways, gaining the weight had helped Summer, if she was open to the lesson, to learn what she needed to learn when she lacked the skills and experience to learn it any other way. Just as it had for me.

I want you to list the lessons that weight gain or weight dissatisfaction have given you. How has your negative body image forced you to wake up? What has it brought to your attention?

Now, how has your situation motivated you to change? How has it opened your eyes to the importance of self-care? What have you learned from your negative body image that could help you become positive on the rest of your journey through life?

Because once you are willing to give your body credit, you can finally take responsibility for it. . . .

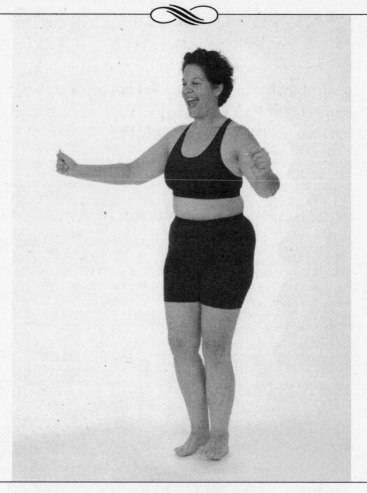

ROBERTA

Height: 5'9" • Weight: 204 pounds • Age: 47

Body Thoughts: *I have been on a seven-year pity party,
and the party is over. I have betrayed my body and now
I am willing to accept it.*

CHAPTER 9

How Do I Take My
First Step?

As we've discovered, most of us have such unrealistic expectations of ourselves that disappointment is a normal feeling and one that, with much regret, we live with on a daily basis. It seems like we can never accomplish all we want when we want it. I understand. I tried that path many times, but it never gave me the results or the peace I yearned for. Instead, it just fueled my fears and fanned the flames of resentment, giving me permission to give up on myself over and over again.

But I've learned to do things a little differently. I have learned to take things one step at a time. By committing to taking just one step at a time, I am learning how to integrate my new behaviors into my life rather than trying to dump my entire life and make up a new one on the spot.

In the beginning, I felt a little lazy and wanted to beat myself up for not doing enough. But thank goodness, I learned my lesson and knew that if I was calling myself a name, it was only fear calling me to do more. With my commitment to freedom firmly in place, I didn't listen and decided to take one step. A small step for some, but an enormous step for me. It was the beginning of my newfound path of living a life free of shame.

Are you ready to take your first step? Here it is: Water.

You've heard it a thousand times before . . .

"Our bodies are made up of more than 70 percent water."

"You've got to drink more water!"

"You can never be too rich, too thin, or drink enough water!"

"Are you drinking your water?"

"In order to be healthy, you MUST ingest eight to ten glasses a day of water!"

Maybe you, like me, have become an expert at resisting your body's need for hydration—justifying that, at some other time, you'll figure out how to get all that liquid down your gullet and into your system. Next month. Next year. Sometime when it's more convenient and your stomach's not so full of pizza and sandwiches and cereal and cake and stuff.

You're willing to stop (or at least slow down) the rationalization that, as along as you're drinking something, you're doing okay—even if that something is loaded with sweeteners and chemicals. You know you should be drinking less soda and more water. Or just more water in general. But where do you begin? (By the way, this doesn't mean you're off the hook with your other unhealthy habits, but we've got to start somewhere.)

As usual, my transformation to healthier habits involved my best friend, Marta.

Marta was the first person in my life who ever asked me how I was feeling physically. We'd been friends for several years when she started asking me how I was feeling. *Huh?* How odd. Well, fine, I'd say. But that was never good enough for Marta. She would ask the same question over and over again—until I told her the truth. Come to think of it, my knee was aching. My hip hurt. Oh, and my head was pounding for the third time this week. I had been doing my best not to feel or acknowledge these little aches and pains because they made me feel like a wimp, a whiner, a loser. Admitting to anyone, including myself, that I wasn't physically strong and capable would mean that I didn't have mastery over the one area of life you'd think I'd be able to control . . . my own self!

Then again, I don't know where I got the idea that I should have control over my body, because in the family I grew up in, bodies didn't exist. I was raised in a household where emotions, let alone bodily functions, were never discussed. That was just way too intimate, too problematic.

My mother never asked me how I was feeling, so when Marta did, I almost fell off my chair. What kind of a question was that? My mother never asked me how I felt about my body as it was beginning to transition into womanhood. My father never discussed the difference between a bicep muscle and a calf muscle. The underlying messages I was taught: *If you break your leg, you deal with it. If you burn your hand, you suck it up. Slip and fall? You're just a klutz, dummy, so get up and dust yourself off.* There was no patience shown toward anyone who couldn't keep up. And absolutely no complaining was allowed.

My grandmother, Mayme, carried a cane for as long as I can remember. With her silver hair in a bun and a limp in her leg, Grandma would walk a mile every day to the long-term care facility where my grandfather lay critically ill for months on end with various ailments, including heart disease. I never saw my grandmother cry about the fact that her husband of sixty years was laid up indefinitely. I never heard my mother ask her how she was handling it all—if she was all right. Grandma and I never had a conversation about her hopes and fears and what lay ahead, for herself, her marriage, or any of us, for that matter.

As a child, the overriding message I received loud and clear was that our bodies were necessary, but ignorable. Emotions surrounding our bodies, how they age and eventually die, were unimportant at best, and pretty much taboo.

Because my body was irrelevant, deciding to care for it by simply drinking water was a huge first step for me. The water was Marta's idea. Her subtle coaxing began during one of our many lunches where she wouldn't let me leave the table until I downed just one glass of room-temperature water. To get her off my back, I did it. But that only encouraged her. She started asking me how much water I drank on our regular evening phone calls. My usual answer was "I don't know," but with Marta's prompting, I found myself traipsing into the kitchen to grab a glass of water so I could drink it while we were on the phone.

During what I call "Marta's water obsession," I drank it to appease her. I didn't really believe that drinking eight glasses of *anything* would add value to my life. I had been getting along fine. Everyone's got aches and pains, right? Well, not necessarily, as I found out when I started asking around. Not everyone has sore joints or backaches or debilitating headaches. While it's true that I was getting by and probably wasn't facing any life-or-death issues anytime soon, I knew in my heart that I wasn't thriving. My quality of life was less than it could be. Marta knew it too; that's why she kept pushing. That's what led me to start drinking the good stuff. If nothing else, it was worth a shot.

Eight Glasses a Day

Around this same time, I had a client named Cheryl who hated drinking water. "I resent the fact that there are so many damn rules to being healthy," she complained in one of our first sessions. *Me too, honey*, I thought, but I also knew that I couldn't be an effective coach for Cheryl if I didn't come up with a way to motivate her away from sodas and toward healthy habits. I needed to find a strategy to let her know she was slowly poisoning her system, even though she didn't believe that to be true. What made me so certain? What gave her away? I could see that Cheryl was in need of some inner cleansing because her eyes lacked sparkle. Her skin was dry, ruddy. Her energy was low, and frankly, she often had bad breath. Looking across the couch at her image, I could suddenly see that Cheryl's system was thirsty for water. Or cleansing, which I assumed would come through a higher intake of water. Was it possible that others saw similar symptoms in me?

That made me nervous. So I started doing a little research. I love the work of Jeffrey S. Bland, Ph.D., who says in his book *Genetic Nutritioneering* that, "Water is an essential nutrient that not only hydrates the body but also provides the proper cellular environment so cells can engage in biochemical reactions associated with gene expression, protein synthesis, and metabolic function." So maybe his wording isn't too sexy, but the point is, if your cells aren't hydrated, survival of the fittest will be reserved for someone else's family. Dr.

Bland recommends, as do many doctors and scientists, that we drink eight to ten glasses of water a day. Who am I to argue with a smart and respected doctor?

So I tried drinking the recommended amount. With some great results, I might add. My eyes looked brighter—my skin did, too. I had fewer sugar cravings and even thought I might be sleeping better. But it wasn't easy. Not just because I'm busy with work and life and exercising, but because, ironically, I'm also busy *eating*. I don't know about you, but when I'm eating, I don't want to fill my stomach with a lot of liquid. I heard once that drinking liquids with your meals actually dilutes your digestive enzymes and makes it harder for your body to get energy from your food and burn off the excess calories. That not only made sense to me, but that's how it *feels*. I feel bloated if I drink too much with my food, no matter how pure the beverage. But I also feel less bloated if I drink plenty of water during the day—without food.

I was mulling over this drinking eight glasses a day issue one afternoon when I was having lunch at Marmalade Café on Ventura Boulevard. I looked down at my salad and thought, "But I'm eating lettuce and apples and carrots and melon all the time, and they're FILLED with water. Does *that* count?" It's then that I stumbled across the concept of "natural hygiene," a way of eating that's been around for more than a century and recommends eating, not drinking, a diet of predominantly raw foods. Water-rich foods. Apparently, according to natural hygienists (and even *Fit for Life*), the more water you *eat* in the form of unprocessed fruits and vegetables, the less you need to drink.

The reason I think this issue is important is because of the emotional element underlying the "drink eight glasses" rule. I know I'm not the only one who's been walking around with "water guilt"—

that nagging daily, even hourly, worry that I'm deficient and starving my body of its most vital need. I thought I wasn't disciplined enough. Didn't love myself enough. That I was being selfish toward my cells! Even though I've developed all sorts of little tricks to help me reach my eight glasses, sometimes I just forget.

It Really Does Work

So where does that leave you—the average person just trying to learn how to take care of and make peace with the body she's got? As we discussed earlier, it's time to learn to listen to your body and trust yourself. That applies here too. I'm a Life Coach, not a doctor, so rather than trying to teach you all of the "scientific" facts on health (which isn't even possible), my intent is to get beyond the science to the underlying emotional reasons we do what we do. That's where the greatest change can originate.

You can get lazy when it comes to drinking water, right? Just admit it. Experts can argue whether or not we need four glasses per day or eight, and if you can eat it rather than drink it, but some people don't eat or drink any! Or they have one glass throughout the day while eating very few fruits and vegetables. Their diet, as some would say, is made up of mostly "dead" foods that leave them feeling sluggish and increasingly hungry due to nutritional deficiencies. It only takes common sense to realize that since your body is 70 percent water (as you age it can get as low as 50 percent), you're stacking the odds against yourself by having a diet that consists of 10 percent water. You do the math.

I have clients who tell me they get thirsty all the time (almost always in the morning), but that they're too lazy or too busy to make sure they've got enough fresh water in the house. One woman I know works at home and sleeps upstairs. She keeps her water in the kitchen downstairs, but wakes up several hours before her family gets up to start her paperwork in her office. She's never as thirsty as she is in the morning, but she's too preoccupied with work to go downstairs and get a glass of water. So she doesn't drink in the morning. Say what? Of course she feels major guilt about her "laziness" all day long, because once she starts eating, she never seems to drink any water. I gave her some light homework. "Just grab two small bottles of water with you on your way upstairs each night," I said. "Drink the first after you brush your teeth when you wake up, and the second an hour later at your desk, before you go down for breakfast."

Ta da! It worked like a charm! She not only feels healthier and "cleaner" and more "regular" (something she thought only came from her coffee intake with breakfast), but she no longer feels bad about herself for being "lazy."

While everyone's different, you will know what's right for you if you take the time to listen to what your body is telling you. If you're thirsty, instead of grabbing a piece of gum or a chocolate bar (or God forbid, a bag of chips), see if a glass of water or an apple or a handful of baby carrots does the trick instead. Take the time to discover your unique water needs.

Water is vital to my ultimate health and well-being—whether it comes from bottles or raw foods or both. I'd like to say that I became miraculously aware of my body and started a rigorous program of water drinking and self-love overnight. Not so. Marta began asking me how I felt physically more than ten years ago, at a time when drinking water was practically a foreign concept to me. Now I line up small bottles of water in my office at the *Starting Over* house to remind myself to drink. I've asked my office assistant to say the word "water" to me throughout the day, and it helps. And when I'm not in the mood to drink, I order a salad or eat an apple or a slice of watermelon.

Learning to live with the body I have has been one of the most difficult and rewarding experiences of my life. Being friends with my body constantly challenges my perceptions and points out my humanity. I still get impatient and want to be an energetic size 4 without any hassles. But I've also learned that there's no free lunch—my physiology won't perform to its optimum unless I give it what it needs.

A rumbling stomach, an aching knee, a strained back—all are warning signals that something's up. My lack of water was sagging my skin and stuffing up nature's natural elimination process. When I made the commitment to drink water on a regular basis and eat a higher-water-content diet, I began experiencing a relationship that I didn't know existed. My body and I began to talk to each other. Or should I say, I began to listen.

All along I had thought that I was in charge of my body, but in fact, it was the other way around. My body determines my capacity to move around in this world. I can either help it or hinder it. My daily habits were hurting me and, eventually, would have been the death of me. Drinking water and eating lots of fruits and vegetables began to change all that. Without even knowing it, my journey to good health had begun.

Beyond the Eight Glasses

Drinking water was the first step I took in taking responsibility for my body. And then the oddest thing happened. As I drank and *ate* more water, I noticed that I was less bloated before, during, and after "that time of the month." Instead of gaining the usual five pounds, I was barely moving the scale. This new regime was working so well that I wanted to change other habits too. I wanted to learn about everything. Vitamins seemed the next logical, or should I say, easy, step. I wasn't yet ready to hit the gym or give up my desserts, but I could swallow a vitamin or two. I was assured by my health-care professional that due to the increased stress in our environment and decreased nutrition in our food supply, almost everyone can benefit from taking a multivitamin. Immediately upon doing so, I had more energy during the day and slept better at night. Taking a basic vitamin tablet has also reduced my susceptibility to colds by boosting my immune system. Every day I make sure I take the daily recommended C, B's, and D, plus some calcium. It gives me peace of mind knowing that although my food may not have all the nutrients I need, I am doing what I can to make sure my body gets what it needs.

Two small steps implemented over a twelve-month period altered my relationship with my body. For the first time I became conscious of it through caring for it and not belittling it. Are you ready to make a small change? Taking responsibility for your health is one of the first steps in learning to accept, and eventually like, your body.

The better you take care of your body, the better your body will take care of you.

Making a commitment to eat and drink plain ol' H_2O meant keeping track of it, and being regimented has never been my strong suit. Before I took responsibility for my body and how I felt about it, I had never kept any sort of food diary or exercise journal. In my mind, what was the point if it would tell me something I wasn't ready to hear? Except one thing: I was asking my clients to keep such journals and it was working. Who was I to say that I didn't need to practice what I preached?

Even knowing all the good drinking water does, I still have to check off the boxes marked "water" in my Daily Training Manual, otherwise I will forget to give myself credit for every glass I sip and gulp. And I don't want to forget, because giving myself credit builds my confidence—confidence I want more of when it comes to my body.

I urge you to follow my example and place eight small water bottles (or four medium or two large) on your kitchen counter. At the end of the day, check to see how well you hydrated yourself.

Don't forget to hold yourself accountable. Decide now how you will keep track of your water. Will you put a check mark in your daily calendar that holds all your to-dos and business appointments? Will you hang a special calendar near your refrigerator? What about doing what I do and counting your water bottles at the end of the day to see how well you are paying attention to your body's needs? What are you willing to do to take this first step?

What if you are feeling that you are drinking enough water now and don't need this exercise? Keep track of your water for a week, just to check. I know too many people who think they are drinking enough water when in fact they are drinking all right, but it ain't water.

Being accountable for your health is one of the most powerful gifts you can give yourself. So let's be sure to acknowledge ourselves for what we are willing to do each day, what risks we are willing to take. How do you do that? Through your daily acknowledgments.

Most of us have a difficult time patting ourselves on the back for the work we are doing. We have plenty of reasons why we should be better, more, or different, so there is always some reason why we shouldn't give ourselves credit. Well, today is the day I would like you to practice doing just that: giving yourself credit.

Your Exercise

How do you give yourself credit? It's simple. Just fill in the blanks.
Today, I acknowledge myself for:

1. _____
2. _____
3. _____
4. _____
5. _____

Acknowledge yourself anytime you are doing something out of the norm, stretching outside of your comfort zone. Doing something like increasing your water intake may seem like a no-brainer, but it isn't. It's work, and I want you to acknowledge yourself for your effort and willingness to change.

Why five? Because I want you to search for ways that you are risking and growing. Acknowledgment is a simple exercise, but very tough to do. If you are a people-pleaser or a perfectionist, it may feel like your toughest assignment to date.

Let me give you a few examples:

Today, I acknowledge myself for carrying water in my car.
Today, I acknowledge myself for setting the alarm on my watch and taking a sip of water every hour on the hour.

*Today, I acknowledge myself for being willing to put eight
small bottles on my desk, even though I felt silly.*
*Today, I acknowledge myself for choosing watermelon, a
water-dense fruit, as my sweet treat rather than a slice of
apple pie.*
*Today, I acknowledge myself for putting a bottle of water near
my bed so I can be sure to take sips before I fall asleep and
then, first thing in the morning.*

Those are just some of the acknowledgments I have given myself
over the past year. Notice how acknowledgments are all about stretching. You do not acknowledge yourself for something you already do
with ease. And yes, you may acknowledge yourself for the same
thing more than once in a week, but please, attempt to acknowledge five different things every day.

Acknowledging yourself goes beyond water. This is an exercise I
want you to use every day to build up your self-confidence, take responsibility for your growth, and give yourself credit where credit is
due. Don't worry. You won't get a big head. Rest assured that because you have put yourself down for so long, that it isn't impossible.

This is a simple, but life-changing first step. If you are willing to
do this, imagine what your future could hold. For me, drinking water and acknowledging myself for it gave me the courage to take on
something a little more daunting. . . .

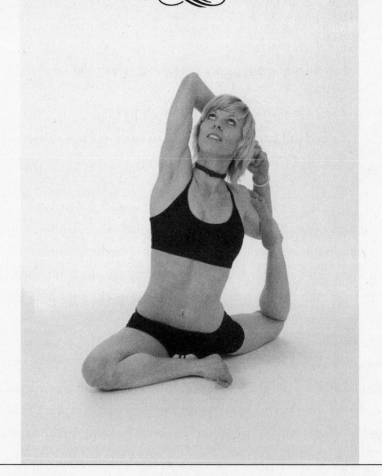

RENEE

Height: 5'7" • Weight: 113 pounds. • Age: 31

Body Thoughts: *Many times I feel like a fraud. People compliment me on my shape and how fit I am. If they only knew that many days I barely have enough energy to make it through the day because of migraines.*

Favorite Exercise: *Yoga saved my life!*

CHAPTER 10

What's the Point
of Exercising?

We've all heard the stats. Exercise is the number one thing you can do to improve your health. Getting that blood moving through your veins through physical activity is important for circulation, elimination, and your metabolism.

Housework is nice and so is running errands, but they're not enough for optimal health. We need our muscles to work every day in order to keep ourselves healthy and happy. Muscles that aren't used lose their tone and become powerful fat makers. Here's what Robert K. Cooper, Ph.D., says in his book *Low-Fat Living*. "When your muscles start to atrophy—which is literally what happens when you begin to lose muscle tone—the signal that tells those muscles to produce fat-burning enzymes gets steadily fainter. As that happens, the easier it becomes for dietary fat to be stored as body fat. And once stored, it's likely to stay there, rather than being released into the bloodstream for burning in your increasingly less active muscles." Whew! Sign me up. I don't want that to happen to me. . . .

But I never learned to exercise. My mother never exercised. In fact, I never actually saw anyone exercising for anything other than a sport while I was growing up. What did I learn? That exercise is done in spurts to achieve a goal but never done consistently or for anything more than a means to an end.

So I never engaged in long-term physical activity. It was always for a limited amount of time to reach a very specific goal: reducing my body fat for my high school reunion, lowering my cholesterol before my next doctor's visit, practicing dribbling for a better spot on the basketball team. It was never a lifestyle choice, never done for the sheer enjoyment of it, never for anything but to get my body in that perfect shape so I could get something or avoid something else.

Why bother to exercise? I thought. *It doesn't stick anyway. I mean, you have to keep doing it over and over again, so it clearly doesn't work.* I lost weight just to gain it all back. I got my cholesterol down to watch it go right back up. I seriously thought once I exercised for a certain number of days and reached my goal, I would keep that change forever while lying on the couch for the rest of my life. Sadly, that's what most people think.

Out of my frustration and a deep sense of failure, I would let my body go again. Since nothing stuck, I thought I might as well give up. I would let my tummy bulge (sit-ups took too long to work anyway), lose muscle tone in my thighs (if I didn't run or walk for a week it looked like I never walked a day in my life, so what's the point), and watch as the elasticity in my upper arms would begin to droop (there is no such thing as spot reducing—even though all the magazines say so).

My experience of exercise was no experience at all. I just did what I did when I did it, and if I didn't get what I wanted, I gave up for a really good reason: *It didn't work*. Right?

My Champion Season

My weight trainer says that it takes a person five to seven years of devotion to a sport to reach his or her genetic potential. Heck, I never devoted my life to *anything* for that long. I mean, who wants to wait around for five to seven years to see results? That was my thinking. Back then, I wanted quick results for the littlest possible effort.

And that's the seduction. That's what we are promised when we read about the latest exercise craze. Have you ever read an advertisement that said, "Try now and in five years you will see results"? Nope. Me neither. What I do see is "Twenty Days to a Tight Tummy" or "Ten Minutes a Day to Your Dream Body." Hmpf. No wonder we think that we must not be doing something right when we make any effort at all. No wonder we have completely unrealistic expectations of what our body should be doing based on our workout level.

Unless you have made health your number one priority or trained for a sporting event like a marathon, you probably have little idea what it takes to be devoted to your body, your health, your life. Unless your body is at the top of your priority list and your exercise routine is an important event in your day, it's hard to really know what devotion looks like. And in some ways, that's what I am asking you to do. Unless you are really willing to see exercise as a life-saving and life-enhancing activity, it will just end up being another thing on your to-do list. And by no means will that get you in touch with your body and help you get on with your life. I didn't even know what the benefits to moving my body really were even though I had read all the books, tried all the latest workout equipment, and even lifted weights and worked out off and on for years.

So what if I told you that you'll have the best body you can have, but it might take you five to seven years to attain it? Would you stick with it? Do you think you could keep up the consistency and commitment necessary to reach your ultimate body goals? And what if I told you that part of "feeling fat" is stress-related and that sleep, recovery, and rest are an important part of the solution?

Even as little as a year ago, I don't know if I could have answered in the affirmative. I hadn't had results, not the kind I wanted. Sure, I felt better. I was moving my body more than most and choosing food that came directly from the ground rather than a package. But it wasn't until I took on exercise as a way of life, not a season, that my definition of commitment really changed. The results have been stellar.

I heard once that every athlete has a "championship season" — a time in his or her sporting "career" where everything comes together and they can do no wrong. Some people call it being in the flow. I call it the thing I grew up dreaming about.

My father was a sports addict; he loved sports more than just about anything. Definitely more than me. I remember thinking that my role, as the middle of three girls, was to be the boy my father wanted. So I tried sports. Lots of sports.

Softball was a disaster. I couldn't hit a ball unless it was bigger than a beach ball. Soccer? Forget it. Getting kicked in the knees was never much fun. Next, I tried basketball. I liked it all right, but the sport didn't like me. During my first year playing in the ninth grade, I accumulated more splinters from the bench than points on the board. But I was determined. It was my third sport, and I thought this might be the way to get my dad to love me.

All of my life, when I told people that my father hated me, they always said something like, "Don't be silly, Rhonda. Your father loves you. He just doesn't know how to show it." It made me wonder if I was crazy. How could it be so hard for a father to show love for his own child? Plenty of dads were able to love their daughters—I'd see them in the stands at games, cheering for their girls, and hugging them when the game was through. Was I just paranoid? Was I too negative? Still, I knew in my gut that he wished I'd never been born. A kid knows these things. You can feel it.

When I was twelve years old, I was walking up the stairs from our basement, and my father was walking down the stairs. He asked me to do something that I no longer remember, and I made some smart-mouthed comment. I'll never forget the look he gave me. His eyes became real squinty and his grin turned into a grimace—I could see right then and there that he was mad, and you did not want to get my dad mad.

I ran for my life, through the kitchen, through the dining room, down the hallway, and into my room. I shut the door to my bedroom as fast as I could, knowing that it wouldn't stop him, but hoping it would slow him down. I got on my bed, laid on my back, and put my arms and legs up for a fight. He slammed through the room, jumped on top of me, and put his hands around my neck and squeezed hard. I could feel the rage in his grip. I put my hands on his and tried to push him off, but he was too strong for me. I was trying to suck in air, any air, and when that didn't happen, I started to imagine how my mother would find me. How my dad would be sorry. How my sisters would miss me. I was feeling dizzy and started to resign myself to dying, so I let go and just laid there hoping it would end quickly. That was when my baby sister Linda ran through the door, jumping on her bed and begging him to stop. I can still hear her chant, "Don't kill Rhonda, Daddy. Don't kill Rhonda." I don't know how many times she said it; all I know is that he eventually stopped. He just got off of me and walked away. It was never talked about, and nothing was ever done. I was simply left knowing that my sister saved my life, and it confirmed that my daddy didn't love me.

So you can imagine my father's dismay at having a bench-warmer for a daughter. He never came to watch any of my basketball games. If you had asked him, he probably would have said, "When she gets off the bench, then I'll come," but I can't say for sure. Maybe he was embarrassed that his daughter couldn't make the first string on the basketball team. Maybe he couldn't stand the thought of seeing me sitting there on the bench while the other kids made baskets. I don't know. All I know was that while I was sitting on the sidelines, no one from my family ever came to cheer me on.

Since basketball wasn't going well, I thought I would audition to become a cheerleader. They're athletes, right? And they get to look good and are definitely popular. In my small school, cheerleaders were a big deal, cheering for everything—basketball, hockey, and football. If I made it, I'd be the female version of a stud because I'd get to wear that cool, prestigious uniform all year round. It was a huge, HUGE thing to be a cheerleader at our school. To me, it was my way out. It was life itself.

I was determined to make it. I knew how to do a cartwheel and I could yell with the best of them. This, I thought, would be my chance. I practiced my cartwheels nonstop. I mastered the splits. Then came the big day: tryouts. It was my turn to go before the judges. My heart was pounding with excitement. Adrenaline was pushing me past my fears. But just before it was my turn, all of my failed athletic attempts began to play a chorus in my brain: *Don't screw up, Rhonda. Don't screw up.* I had just finished acing a cartwheel and a somersault when everything sort of got blurry. I felt like I was falling. And I was. *Hold it, Rhonda,* I thought. *Don't fall now.* But it was too late. In the middle of my splits, my butt was on the gym floor when it was definitely not supposed to be anywhere near it. My attempt at being a cheerleader was a big fat failure. To say the least, I didn't make the team.

My parents didn't see that either. Thank God. I was so embarrassed. I vowed I would never feel that way again. But what I didn't know was that, if I wasn't willing to open myself to feeling that vulnerability, I would never audition for anything, ever. I had created a trap for myself, one that I had to feel my way out of—the very thing I wasn't willing to do.

A funny thing happened after my parents died. I became a better athlete, thanks to my mother. She died on June 15, 1975, at the end of my freshman year in high school. Right before she passed, my mother did something she had never done before—she signed me up for summer sports camps. I'm sure she was trying to figure out a way to patch things up between me and my dad, and she knew that sports would be the answer. That July and August, I kept busy, going from basketball camp to basketball camp. It saved me. It gave me an outlet for my grief. I channeled all of my rage and pain into every dribble drill, every shootout, every run around the track. I was voted the most improved player that summer at camp after camp.

When we got back to school in the fall, I quickly became the leading scorer on the junior varsity team, and before the end of the season, I was called up to the big leagues: varsity.

That was a huge confidence boost and one that I secretly relished.

In retrospect, that was my champion season—the season my layup couldn't miss the net and every point on the board was like sweet revenge. Maybe my father would have finally been proud of me. But he didn't get to see it. He didn't get to watch his middle daughter turn into a jock.

Everyone Needs a Cheerleader

I applaud teachers and coaches so much! When my relatives were too guilt-ridden to face me, my coaches and teachers became my surrogate parents. They supported me and told me that I was doing a good job. I always say that no one can be fearless alone. Everyone needs support. I may have appeared to be happy and successful on the outside, but in reality, I was very much alone and lonely. If it hadn't been for my coaches and teachers standing on the sidelines and praising my efforts, I don't think I'd ever be emotionally capable of coaching others now. I might not even be alive.

What does my childhood trauma have to do with my body image and my relationship to exercise? Everything. For starters, because my father was a sports nut who wouldn't come to see me play sports, I had a strong sense that I was a failure before I had even given myself a shot. If you'll notice, my father had to die before I could excel and feel my power.

Your Exercise

While my case is an extreme case, you might want to take some time to determine what messages you received from your parents and who your cheerleaders have been. Grab a pen and piece of paper, and answer the following questions:

What kind of beliefs do you still hold from your parents or authority figures?

What did people expect of you, and how are you still giving them your power?

What kind of message did you receive about your athletic prowess? Were you encouraged to dance around the garden, to bike to the market down the street, or to skate fast around the rink? Were you told to throw the ball even though you weren't the best catcher, or to play golf even though it took you nine strokes to get it into the cup? Or did you hear "slow down," "be careful, you will get hurt," or "you can't do that?"

The messages we received from our parents influence our entire lives unless we decide to make our opinion, our decisions matter more. We have to decide that we want to see ourselves as an athlete, a jock, an adventure girl before we will decide to give it our all.

I Never Knew

Before I traced my exercise history, I never understood why I couldn't stay with an exercise plan longer than a few months. I'd do really well for two or three months, and then I'd fall into my self-defeating habits and quit. This became really obvious to me when I worked for a goal to lose weight before my twenty-year high school reunion. I was so motivated because I was NOT going to show up weighing 150 pounds. So, I worked out hard for three months, harder than I ever had before. And my prize? A size 6 dress that I slipped into with ease due to my slim weight of 135 pounds. I looked great, and that dress was the skinniest, tightest dress I could find. Mission accomplished. I had a terrific trip and got lots of attention, but it didn't last. I came home, stopped working out, and returned to my "regular" life before exercise. My healthy habits didn't continue past the special occasion because they were event-driven, not a long-term gradual change of lifestyle. No, no, no. It had to happen all at once or I wasn't interested.

At the same time, I also noticed that my interest in healthy habits was a time-of-year thing. Why is it that when September comes around, I'm all motivated, but as soon as the holidays approach, I'm a slug? You know what? This is a big realization, and maybe also a challenge you've experienced: I was still on my old school-year schedule! Back in school, each sport would last between two and three months, and then there would be a break before the next one would start. I was still going for three months, and then still taking my breaks! I ask you: Are you still on your old school-year schedule? If so, it's time to see the pattern and find a new schedule!

I had to find mine. It's called any time, all the time. Let me explain.

My desire to be happy in my own skin, to embrace my body, happened before I ever hit the *Starting Over* house. But once I was working every day in front of the camera, I had no time to add working out to my schedule. I wanted to stay "sweat-free," so if I had an hour break, I couldn't go to the gym and lift weights or grab a few miles on the treadmill. Nope. Not only did I want to look the best I could on camera, I had always judged people who wore makeup in the gym. In the past, makeup in the gym, to me, meant pick-ups, not workouts. I abhorred the desperation I felt the women must be living with if they had to show up looking like that. You can see my dilemma.

So during my first season as the Life Coach on *Starting Over*, I barely made it to the gym. My commitment to exercising had just been added as the third step to my healthy lifestyle routine, after water and vitamins, so I didn't feel the need to be the perfect exercise student. I just got there when I could—usually an average of two to three times a week, sometimes for as little as thirty minutes. *But at least I was doing something*, I told myself. And that was true.

Between the first and second seasons of taping the show, I hired a trainer and started working out in earnest. I liked it. I felt strong, capable, and excited to be experiencing new sensations in my body, to actually have a goal of looking and feeling my best. I wanted that commitment to continue when we began to shoot the second season, but with my rigid rules of "no makeup in the gym" and needing to be "sweat-free," I only had time for minimal workouts. I wasn't happy. I wanted to move my body more than once every three weeks. I wanted to at least do something every other day, but how? It would mean I would have to be willing to break all the rules, let go of all my judgments.

Joining the local gym was tough because now I was the woman who wore makeup to the gym. I was the one who sweated up a storm, went into the dressing room to reapply my makeup, and put the same clothes on that I had worn before the sweat parade. At first, it was a disaster. My hair went flat, my makeup was all matty, and I felt sticky all day long. But then something happened. I liked working out more than looking good. It was the shift I needed.

During the second half of that season, I began to leave the *Starting Over* house and hit the gym whenever I had a break of more than thirty minutes. I would take a walk, do some sit-ups, or attend a spinning class. My hair was a tad flatter than when I started, no matter how much hairspray I used. And yes, my makeup had to be touched up more often than not. But my body loved it.

By the time we began filming the third season, I didn't care about makeup at the gym or putting on clothes after I sweated a bit; what mattered was that I was taking care of myself. It was a huge shift in thinking and it had taken me more than two years of continuous baby steps to reach it, to embrace living a healthy lifestyle.

Now that I look back at my judgments about makeup in the gym, I think about how narrow my mind was, how unsympathetic I could be, and how it just proved how little I knew about commitment.

Your Commitments Matter

Making a commitment to love your body is not just a bunch of words. It is action in motion. You will be called to put your commitment before convenience. You must be willing to place judgments, opinions, and other people's needs second to what is important to you. A commitment means that you must devote a certain amount of time on a daily basis to embody what you value. It means you must live with integrity.

I've found that it's enough to make a commitment just for yourself. Even if no one else cares—if not another soul in the world is watching—do it for *you*. If you reach your goal (to start lifting weights, eat more vegetables, or run a marathon), you have the rest of your life knowing that no one can take it away from you. My parents were taken away from me in an instant, but no one can take away the fact that I became a starter on the basketball team. And nowadays, I'm finding that I'm exercising for the sheer health of it, and that's enough. I had to be willing to put aside my competitive spirit to give up the goal of being skinny or winning races, and to care about myself enough to do so without a reward at the end. I might never win a trophy. I might never lose my last ten pounds. But that's not the point. It's about consistency and commitment and taking care of *me*. I trust that results will happen naturally.

I've discovered that nothing is worth more than honest, hard work and self-care. If I pushed myself for a week or a month, like the old Rhonda used to do, I would only be abusing myself and nothing would ever stick. Not the muscles. Not the weight loss. Not the self-esteem.

As I've said over and over again, if you ignore your body and your needs, they will be heard. Even if your body has to get loud to be heard.

So what will your commitment be? Do you want good health, a long life, a healthy heart? All of those goals take a commitment to move your body on a regular basis. We've all heard it: Use it or lose it, and there is no better example of that cliché than your body.

When you commit to a long-term process, you start noticing fluctuations of your body on a weekly and monthly basis. You'll notice how your hormones affect your weight. You'll notice what foods cause you to retain water, and you'll understand the difference between water weight gain and weight (fat) gain. You'll know the feeling of fat vs. muscle, and you'll understand that the number on the scale has become a mere reference point.

Short-lived goals will never help you build a long-term relationship with your body. Start now to look back at your past, find your patterns, and commit to starting anew. Maybe, if you're like me, your body was a vehicle to get you something, rather than a partner in helping you achieve a healthy life. Remember, no one (including me) can do it alone. You need your body. Your mind is only so good, and can only take you so far. Without a healthy body to feed your mind, you can't reach your potential. You are one unit—a mind/body connection—and you must have integration between your head, your heart, and your body, or you will never reach your genetic potential.

Doing so is easier than you think. It starts with a willingness to look at the past, take healthy action today, and stay the course on a year-round lifestyle schedule (rather than a three-month school schedule).

We have to get beyond the championship season and think of ourselves as champions for life.

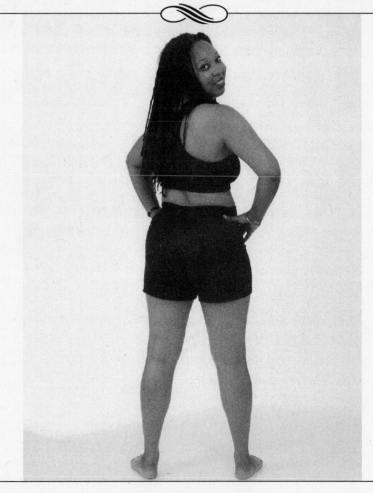

DANA

Height: 5'6½" • Weight: ? • Age: 36

Body Happiness: *Life is too short to be tied to a daily
number on a scale.*

Dieting: *I have never dieted. I don't believe in it, but I decided to
slowly change my body by healthier eating habits.*

Competition: *I think people have too much time on their hands if
they are thinking about my body. I don't think about theirs.*

CHAPTER 11

Am I Fated to Be Fat?

Americans are obsessed with food. That's no big secret. We're famous the world over for our super-sized, overindulgent natures. Just how did we get the distinction of being the fattest populace on the globe?

Turn on the television and you'll see that we have entire television stations devoted to the subject of cooking and feeding our never-ending gustatory fixations. A plethora of gourmet magazines are ready to educate us on the latest and greatest recipes from master chefs. We even have dating services built around introducing potential partners around the dinner table. Food is at the center of our social lives, our fantasies, and our entertainment. We worship the stuff. Food has become our salvation. Our best friend. Our lover. Our on-demand, instant everything—in a cup, in a bowl, on a plate, or from a box.

And yet it's not a pure love. You know what I'm talking about. You love chocolate cake, but you hate yourself for eating three pieces in a sitting. You adore french fries but blame them for being the cause of your oily face or indigestion. Cheese is something you swear you're going to stop eating soon, but then you're cursing out your "cheesy thighs" because you couldn't control yourself at the buffet table. Year after year, as the heat of summer gives way to the subtle chill of fall, you dream about creamy soups and banana breads and wish your grandma were still alive to make her holiday Yule logs.

You're not alone. Most of us are as busy obsessing over food as we are trying to ignore it. We've been dancing to this love/hate tune for years. We pretend we don't need it, get mad at ourselves for being "dependent" on it, and then as soon as our hunger kicks in or an emotion arises that we don't want to face, we absentmindedly shove junk into our systems in an attempt to hurry up the process. We end up abusing food, and ourselves. It makes me wonder, are we fated to be fat?

Your Food Legacy

Food is necessary for our very survival. On Abraham Maslow's hierarchy of needs, food is at the bottom. We need food before we can figure out our passion, accept love, or find our higher purpose. Without food, we will die. And therein lies the paradox. *Food: can't live with it, and can't live without it.*

Because we need food, it becomes a convenient scapegoat. We abuse the thing we must have. It's no wonder we're all so mixed up. No matter how many diet books I've read or recipes I've pored over or nutritionists I've consulted, the reality is that food is confusing. Absolutely perplexing. The food pyramid (which has recently changed, by the way) tells me bread is good for me, but my doctor tells me that wheat is one of the most prevalent undetected allergens around. The Atkins Diet espouses that meat is good for my body, but then *Eat to Live* makes a case for worshipping vegetables, and *Fit for Life* recommends that I limit my meat intake and start my day off with fruit. And then add all the books that deal with emotional eating, like *The End of Diets* or *When Food Is Love*, and it is easy to see why we don't know what to eat, let alone know why we are eating. But eating we still are.

When I was seventeen, I was a big fan of the grapefruit diet. Give it two weeks and a beautiful body would be mine. Forget health. Forget working out. "Give me the body now" was my motto. My senior prom was only two weeks away, and as usual, I didn't feel thin enough. Eating grapefruit every day, all day, took little effort. I didn't have to think about my next meal or count calories or prepare my snacks ahead of time. I just had to eat grapefruits—whole, halved, or freshly squeezed. Ripe, pink, glorious grapefruits. Until my lips itched and cracked and my tongue burned and those grapefruits became the last thing on earth I wanted to look at, much less eat.

I lost five pounds, but I knew this was a short-term fix. I couldn't go the rest of my life as a fruitarian, eating nothing but citrus. I knew next to nothing about healthy living—except for the fact that I wasn't doing it. Health experts? I had never met one. Vitamins? Who knew what to take, or how much. Classes? The only thing taught in my high school that dealt with the topic of food had to do with apple strudel in home economics.

Meanwhile, at home I was learning plenty about food and creating my own personal culinary legacy. Grilled cheese and tomato soup? Yummy. Roast beef, mashed potatoes, and canned corn? Count me in. Burnt pork chops and bottled applesauce? A favorite with the Brady Bunch, so how could it be bad? And for dessert, green Jell-O with shredded carrots. Yum. These are the foods my mother served for our family meals. Mom wasn't much of a cook. Canned vegetables were all we had, and those were rarely green. Iceberg lettuce made an appearance on our kitchen table monthly, whether we liked it or not, with nothing more than a tomato slice on top. And we were sorely lacking in fruit. Once a year my mother bought a box of fresh pears from the local A & P. We would sit in our basement, staring at them until my mother deemed them ready to eat. I would devour them as fast as she would allow. Pears were special. And I learned to get along without. This is my family food legacy.

Most of our legacy has been built around the idea of comfort. When we take risks in our adult lives, we can go back to our "safe" teenage worlds through our food choices. We can attempt to exercise, in our minds, some sort of control over our lives. We can't just quit our jobs, but we *can* cave in to our craving for apple pie à la mode. I can hear the excuses now. "Didn't I just sacrifice another day at a job I hate?" or "My boss would be nothing if I wasn't there, but he's the one who gets all the glory and money."

When those feelings overwhelm us, we feel powerless, out of control, helpless. What better way, easier way, really, to take back our power than doing what *we* want by eating what we want? Food is all about the notion of control. As little kids, that was often the only control we had. Mom couldn't make us eat her fried green tomatoes or cooked carrots or that squashy spinach. She could try, but we still had the ultimate say. We could spit it out. Shut our mouths. Say no really loud. Throw our plate. And generally make our parents' lives miserable if they didn't feed us what we wanted. For most of us, that worked. We did get our way—otherwise, we swore we'd starve instead.

So now we believe that the way to get control over our lives is to control what we put in our mouth. Just like we did when we were little. And in theory, that is true. Control is critical to good health. Making a choice to eat veggies instead of gummy bears takes a certain amount of control. Yet, for most of us, control equals rebelling against what's best, stuffing feelings, denying needs. We yearn to feel "in control" by controlling our food, just like we did when we were little. It appears that food becomes the ultimate acceptable power tool.

Changing Your Food Legacy

Just like me, you have had a food legacy handed down to you generation after generation. What's yours? How do you use your food legacy? Do you use it to belittle yourself after you grab one of the brownies at the bakery because it reminds you of your mom? Or do you consciously choose to make that brownie a meal to stay connected with your loved ones? Or all of the above? Perhaps you rebel against it? Your family's favorite food was homemade pasta and now, you refuse to eat what made you feel safe as a child. You've decided that your mother's weight issues will not be handed down to you. No matter what. Good for you for taking a stand, but make sure you're not cutting off your emotions in the process. Rebellion is another form of prison—you're just picking a different straitjacket.

What do you crave when you, once again, people-please by saying yes when you really want to say no? Do you take back control by telling yourself you deserve that delicious piece of strawberry cheesecake? You eat quickly, so no one sees, and tell yourself it's okay. You had a hard day. How about when you're angry at a friend or frustrated with your boss? Is that the time you want something crunchy and salty, like nachos? What about when you want to feel loved by someone who hasn't given you the time of day? Does reaching for something creamy like ice cream or mashed potatoes fit the bill? If you're like me, on a sad, rainy day, nothing hits the spot like chocolate cake (warmed, with whipped cream), and lots of it.

But the challenge is that in our desire to control, we feel out of control. The minute we put the cheesecake in our mouth, we start berating ourselves. The moment the nachos are washed down with a margarita, we ask ourselves, who cares? And all of a sudden, one transgression becomes an evening of stuffing, shoving, and fighting all our feelings, it seems, at one time. At that point, it almost feels like we have no choice.

I'm all about choice and personal power and motivation. Choice is my middle name. But the possibility of choosing what to eat and when to eat must be done consciously. And to be conscious, we must become aware of our feelings, all our feelings. For most of us, that is not easy to do.

Because the concept of choice, of not giving in to all my fears, doesn't hit home, doesn't make me change—unless I dig deep and become aware of the emotions connected to what *I'm* reaching for. When that food baggage is trailing behind me, I get stuck, and making a choice, a healthy choice, seems nearly impossible. My expertise doesn't feel so expert-like after all. It's then that I have to force myself to do my own exercises. The ones that seem easy when I'm handing them out to others yet are hard when I have to do them myself. But that doesn't scare me anymore. I know that hard equals resistance and resistance equals transformation. So bring it on!

Your Exercise

Grab a piece of blank paper and make three columns. In the first column, write down all your favorite foods as a child. If you don't remember, that's okay. If a vague recollection comes up, trust it. Write it down.
Move on to column two and list your favorite foods as a teenager.
What did you reach for when your friend was mean to you, or you
didn't get asked to the dance by your secret crush? In the third column,
list your favorite foods as an adult. Lastly, circle the foods that repeat
themselves. For example, I wanted chocolate when I was a teenager
and still yearn for it as an adult. *Pizza, pizza, and more pizza* is my
motto when I feel self-pity coming on. Ask yourself: Which foods tran-
scend all ages? What craving have you relied on for more than a year?

Childhood Years	Teenage Years	Adult Years

Congratulations for identifying the foods that are connected to your past and continue to trigger you today. And if no foods repeated themselves, congratulations for knowing that your taste buds are flexible and can change.

Our Core Needs

We all have core needs, and food is one way we use to get our needs met. For instance, I want to feel like I belong. What better way to belong than breaking bread together? That's why eating out is a danger zone for me. If I'm unconscious of how my body feels that day, anything goes. Calories don't count and dessert is a must. Perhaps you want to feel loved. If your mother was like mine and served you toast slathered in butter and strawberry jam, fruit cocktail mixed with whipped cream, and a can of 7Up when you were sick, you probably crave foods that have the same taste and texture when you need some extra attention.

There's nothing wrong with having needs and absolutely nothing wrong with wanting them met. Yet when you're unaware of what your needs are, your food legacy will kick in automatically and determine what you eat and how much. And, like me, you will feel like you absolutely have no choice but to pick up those Krispy Kremes and devour them on the spot.

Because of the deep love I carry for my family—especially my mother—I was trying to honor her food legacy, but I didn't know how to do that and still honor my feelings. Is it possible to do both? Do I need to do both?

I may not need to do both, but I want to do both. But first, I must be clear on what I want my relationship with food to look like and figure out what matters to me when it comes to health. Personally, to do what I do, I must have good health. I could never get up every morning, be focused, present, and loving with the women of the *Starting Over* house if I didn't keep myself centered. My food choices are a big part of that.

So every morning I make sure I eat my veggies and have some protein to make sure my muscles are well fed. If only my food legacy mattered, I would consume cereal every morning for breakfast, just like I did daily growing up. But cereal and only cereal will not get me through my day. I need to go beyond my legacy. The same decision-making criterion is in play the rest of my day.

But when I go to my sister's for the holidays, I indulge in the occasional bowl of cereal in the morning and make sure I have grilled cheese and tomato soup, just like Mom used to make. Sharing the food of my mother with my sisters keeps the memory of my mother alive. But to eat like that all the time would hurt the legacy I am trying to create for myself, a new legacy built on different information, different choices, different commitments.

So instead of feeling bad about our family legacies, let's try to honor them and the feelings that come with them. When we do that, we will have the courage to process our past and face our future making the right choices for ourselves.

Your Food Legacy Diary

It's time to become aware of the meaning behind the foods you eat. It's time to find out what you eat and why. I bet you have kept more food diaries than you would ever care to divulge, but I'm asking you to keep one more. This time I want you to keep track of your food legacy. More than your feelings, I want you to become aware of what is driving your cravings.

I believe it's impossible to eat without attaching some hope to the act, whether it's "I wish I were healthy" or "I want to fit in" or "I want to be loved." My intention is to validate what you need so that you can decide how to fulfill those needs outside of food, rather than letting your cravings decide for you and defeat you. I promise this works. Today I crave vegetables, whereas in the past, my cravings only led me to consume nachos or chocolate cake. I'm living proof that cravings change when you take responsibility for your emotional needs. Sometimes, I still need a bowl of Cheerios just because I miss my mom. *But that's okay because it's just sometimes, instead of three times per day!*

Your Exercise

Most people think they know what they eat all day, but few actually do. It's the difference between our memory and reality: We have a tendency to think we are either doing better or worse than we truly are. Today is the day I want you to take responsibility for how, when, and why you eat what you do. Think of it as an opportunity to build your awareness, giving you the courage and the confidence to make decisions that empower your sense of self rather than sabotage all your good intentions.

As you eat throughout the day, write down the time you eat, your food of choice, any meaning you have attached to it, and whether you are eating for convenience, taste, or health. It's important to write down the time of day to help you discover if your hunger signal is working. But remember, no judgment. Most people don't remember what they eat and rarely bother to figure why they eat. Be patient, loving, and kind to yourself as you uncover your relationship with food.

I created my own version of a food diary that works for me. I place my daily food journals into a three-ring binder for ease. You might want to do the same. Or you might want to incorporate your eating habits into the daily planner you currently use, or pick up a special journal that is just for this exercise. It's up to you. The easier you make it, the more likely you'll do it. And don't forget to keep track of your hunger signals.

Your Hunger Signals

What the heck is a hunger signal? A hunger signal is a sign that your body gives you when your body needs to be replenished with nutrients. What about when your tummy is full? It will give you a full signal when your body is satiated with nutritionally sound food. But you must listen carefully. Learning to differentiate a craving from a hunger signal takes patience. Your tummy may be filled, but it may not have adequate nutrition, so it will continue to crave other foods even though you feel stuffed to the gills.

Most of us deprive our body of the food it needs to run at full throttle, and all that deprivation adds up and leads to gluttony sooner or later. Why do we do it? Because we are starving, literally. Starving for affection. Starving for connection. Starving for satisfaction. And in the process, we end up starving ourselves of nutrients.

A few months ago I decided to quit eating solid foods after 7 P.M. and get to bed at a decent time. I could have a protein-carbohydrate shake if hunger hit, but otherwise, tea and water would be it. It was an eye-opening experience. Before this experiment, if you had asked me what hunger felt like, I would have given you a very detailed description, but in reality, I had no idea.

Most people don't know what their hunger signal feels like

because they eat for convenience and in accordance with a predetermined time schedule rather than eating when they truly are hungry. I didn't discover mine until I was eating nutrition-packed foods at regular intervals. In fact, when I first started experiencing my hunger signal, it came as quite a shock. I thought I always knew the signs of hunger: headache, grumpy disposition, jitters. What I discovered is that those weren't hunger signals, those were withdrawal signals. I was withdrawing from addictive foods such as salt, sugar, and caffeine that were only serving my emotional temperament, not my body. What I realized is that when I was feeling like that, sure I had to eat, but I had to fill my body with foods that perhaps, in the beginning, weren't my first choice. But as I learned, and so will you, if you truly want to live to your genetic potential and be as healthy, loving, and expressive as possible, you must choose foods that satisfy more than your sweet tooth. You must satisfy your body.

I know now that what I thought was hunger wasn't. Instead, it was my unhealthy addiction to nutritionally depleted foods. In the past, if my stomach wasn't full, I had to feed it something. Now I see that what I was doing was just keeping myself stuffed all the time — not answering hunger pangs. No wonder I always felt bloated and disgusting. I gave my stomach no breathing room.

When I began to practice my new commitment of protein-carbohydrate shakes only after 7 P.M., I felt a lightness in my abdomen and my bloating went away. Now, on those occasions when I work late at the *Starting Over* house, I do eat solid foods after 7 P.M., but they're healthy foods, like a thick, juicy piece of salmon that contains healthy fats and a good dose of protein, along with some high-fiber multi-colored veggies. During those times, I know I need more nutrients to stay present while I am coaching those long hours. I do not deprive myself because depriving myself is feeding my fear of *I'll never be thin enough*. I want to leave that fear behind—the fear that there is something wrong with me and that something is stopping me from being thin.

When I eat out of habit, at a preset time or because of cravings, I am eating for the wrong reasons. I'm eating because I have nothing to do, or because food has been placed in front of me, or because I have the urge to stuff myself to stave off some emotion I'm afraid to feel. Now I try to eat what my body needs rather than focusing on what everyone else is eating. That hasn't always been easy, but it has been enlightening and empowering. It's given me another way to take care of myself in a loving, nurturing way that heals my heart as well as my body. It is a powerful way that I tell myself I am worthy.

The truth is, many of our cravings happen because of the poor nutritional value that resides in our food. Our body is just trying to get its needs met, and when it feels deprived, it shouts for something different or just more. Poor nutrition is a worldwide epidemic; crops are no longer rotated; soil is rarely given a chance to regain nutrients; crops are sprayed with anything and everything that will make them grow faster and be more disease resistant. Our crops are harvested at an alarming rate, a rate beyond what nature intended, and the food we eat isn't nurturing us as it used to. As a nation, we're starving nutritionally yet packing on the pounds, trying to feed ourselves in our quest to feed physically as well as emotionally.

Taste, Health, or Convenience

In Leon Rappoport's enlightening book *How We Eat*, he writes that people choose the food they eat based on three criteria: taste, health, or convenience. For most of us, those three criteria conflict with each other on a regular basis. And that's where confusion enters the picture. You know you want to be healthy, but your husband has been out of town all week and the kids are driving you crazy, so you go with convenience. Or you are attracted to a guy at work and he is dating someone, a size 2, so your health commitment goes out the window as you scream silently to yourself, "What's the use!?"

Eating that organic salad filled with broccoli, pine nuts, and bite-size tomatoes may be healthy and even tasty, but usually it isn't so convenient. Organic restaurants aren't on every street corner of America, and hormone- and pesticide-free vegetables aren't always easy to come by. If your shopping is dictated by convenience, a high level of health may be compromised.

What about the fast food that *is* on every corner? It's convenient, but it's also laden with artery-hardening oil and fats, thus compromising the requirement of health.

And the race for exquisite taste? Who has time to spend hours in the kitchen creating a scrumptious gourmet meal?

Just how is a girl supposed to focus on her healthy lifestyle when all of these foods are competing for her attention? That's usually when our food legacy takes over. Whenever confusion ensues and our commitment to a healthy way of eating isn't in the forefront of our minds, the foods that have meaning to you will win every time.

How are you starving yourself? What are you dying to feel, to experience, to have? What are you so deprived of you don't even know you want it anymore? What nutrients are you lacking because your comfort foods have taken over?

As we've discussed previously, no one ever taught me to look at my emotions or my physiology with any real interest, so I just kept on eating—hoping to fill the hole left by my father's harshness, my parents' fighting, and the fact that our family life felt anything but secure.

You are not fated to be fat. That's the ultimate excuse. What you are fated to be, according to your genetics, your soul, and your heart, is a magnificent, vibrant person who is worthy of health, well-being, and self-care. Who has the power to choose vegetables over sugar because she wants to, because she can. A woman who knows what she needs because she has decided to listen to her body rather than deprive it, ignore it, or betray it.

Food is truly under your control. You can choose to eat for comfort from your past or decide that true comfort will come from knowing the difference between cravings and a hunger signal. Do not settle for the illusion of control and false comfort. Choose instead to decide your body's fate by deciding what you will feed it and when. You have more control over your body than you think you do.

So I urge you to take back your body by taking true control over your food. And sometimes, if you are going to heal your food issues, you need to learn other ways to nurture yourself. . . .

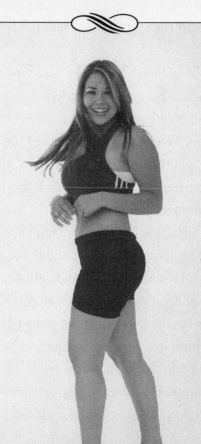

EDEN

Height: 5'5" • Weight: 126 pounds • Age: 30

Body Thoughts: *I think I look foxy in the mirror. I am comfortable, but getting to this place has been a slow and steady journey.*

Diets: *I had tried them all before I figured out that self-love is the key.*

Body Motto: *My body is beautiful, life-giving (two children), and I am grateful for it.*

CHAPTER 12

How Can I Open My Life to Nurturing a Healthy Lifestyle?

My grandparents are from the old country, Finland. They lived through WWI, the Depression, WWII, Korea, and Vietnam. Complaining was not an option. But neither was self-care. There was no time to take a bubble bath with Epsom salts or to light a candle and contemplate your existence. You had to work twenty-four hours a day just to survive. My grandparents did survive, but that survival handed down a legacy of struggle.

Growing up in my family, there was no time for taking leisurely afternoon naps or lounging on the sun porch reading your favorite magazine. Words like *self-care* or *nurture* were considered indulgent, selfish. If you actually had time to take care of yourself, then you had time to help someone else. I remember cutting my hand on a broken glass while washing dishes. My mother tried to stop the bleeding, but once she realized she couldn't, we went to the emergency room. We immediately came back home—just in time to finish my homework. If I fell off my bike, I still got myself home, or else. Sure, I learned resilience and perseverance, and gained a strong work ethic, but it took decades to learn how to give myself a break once in a while. And it took more time to learn the difference between self-love and self-centeredness. A delicate balance for sure, but one that everyone should embrace if we are ever going to truly experience compassion for others and ourselves.

This chapter might be the most difficult chapter for some. It will feel like death to the people-pleasers, perfectionists, and the givers of the world. To some it will feel like a sin. But if you are going to embrace your body, if you truly want it to be a friend rather than a foe, then you will have to take care of it.

What is self-care? What does it mean to nurture your body, mind, and spirit? And what good will it do you? Well, let me answer the last question first. It will do you a world of good.

Money Doesn't Grow on Trees

When I was growing up in Duluth, Minnesota, money was scarce in my family. If my sisters and I asked for anything, my father would tell us in no uncertain terms that money "doesn't grow on trees." And if something had any life left in it, you had to use it until it died. A new bike when the old one still worked? The answer would be a definite no.

After hearing no week after week, month after month, and year after year, I finally quit asking. I understood that being a team player in a house filled with chaos was the best thing to be. I didn't expect much because I knew three things: a) My parents were "Depression babies," having been born at the tail end of the hardest economic time in the history of our country, and they had been raised with little themselves, b) One day I would make my own money—lots of it—and I'd be free to spend as I pleased, and c) You can't get blood from a turnip.

I drew the line, however, when it came to my bedspread.

"Honey," my mother said one day while looking at the JCPenney catalog, "would you like to choose your very own bedspread?" I could hardly believe my ears. Was she serious? I couldn't flip through the pages fast enough. I had shared a double bed with my two sisters until I was almost eight years old, but after much cajoling from Mom, my father gave in and built an upstairs addition to our modest two-bedroom, one-bathroom home. And that meant I would have, for the first time, at age twelve, my *own* room. The thought of sleeping in a bed of my own made me feel like a princess, and frankly, I didn't care how much that bedspread was going to cost: I wanted it and I wanted it now! It meant independence. It meant that I was growing up.

I decided on a soft green one with matching fringe. Plain. Simple. But all mine. That was the beginning of what I call my "bedroom ownership" phase. I may not have been able to tell my mother what kind of carpeting to buy, or what color I wanted painted on my walls, but I had my own room and the simple freedom to choose this one aspect of my room's décor. After the bedspread's arrival, each time I walked through my bedroom door, one glance at it made me smile ear to ear. That gorgeous green material reminded me on a daily basis that freedom and independence and a place to call my own weren't just a far-off wish.

What does this story have to do with my body or your body? Plenty! Every day we create the environment in which our bodies must live, breathe and, hopefully, thrive. My bedspread was more than a bedspread. It was a self-esteem tool, giving me a chance to take responsibility for my happiness. In a small way, a simple item was helping me find out who I was, what I wanted, and where I was going.

I still remember cleaning up the sawdust from my bedroom floor before I put down my new bedspread. I wanted the room to be perfect before I added the finishing touch, the touch that was mine and mine alone. I was so proud.

Consider for a moment where you live. Right now. What does the room you're in this very minute look like? Is it clean? Is the painting finished, or do you still have to touch up the trim? Is there unfolded laundry bunched up in the corner, or are fresh-cut flowers from your garden sitting on the table in front of you?

What is *your* green bedspread? For you, it might be the photograph of the ocean you've always wanted or the desk you think is too expensive, or simply the act of taking the time to organize and file away the stacks of papers you see piled up around the room. Regardless, the environment that surrounds you directly impacts how you wake up in the morning, how you fall asleep at night, and every moment in between.

Decorate, for Health's Sake

Choosing to really occupy your space and make it yours is a testament to your willingness to own all of your parts. If you look at your home as a metaphor, what do you think it means that you hate your drab curtains? In pretending that they don't matter to your self-esteem, what could you be denying about your hatred for your stomach, or your thighs? What about those white walls staring at you while you're lying in bed? Do you really think it's possible that your disdain for them doesn't affect your dream state? What about the sterile office you have yet to make your own?

Some of you have an excuse: "Yeah, but this isn't where I want to stay!" I get it. The fact is, however, you *are* living where you're living, no matter if it's for a week or a year or a decade. Whether it's a mansion, a two-story duplex, a studio apartment, or a friend's basement you're living in, you can begin making the space your own right now.

Where do you start? By telling yourself that you are taking responsibility for your life. Period. Your life isn't hanging in limbo somewhere, on hold for when you get the perfect house or the ultimate husband to go along with that house. Your life is happening *right now*.

It can be hard to stay focused on your life when everyone else's life looks so much better than yours. In Los Angeles it is extremely easy to get caught up in trying to keep up with the Joneses and the Smiths and the Lees. I heard once that there are 50,000 millionaires living in the city proper, and whether or not that's still accurate, the bigger-than-life energy of the city is palpable and pulsates through your very cells, pushing you to achieve.

I want to be rich and famous so that I'll never have any more worries, I used to think. I laugh at that naïveté now. Everyone who's ever watched any number of Hollywood biographies knows how ridiculous that thinking is, but when I was young, it was a common belief that notoriety and stacks of cash brought total freedom. To be honest, even up until a few years ago, I still held tight to some of that idealism. I hadn't yet tasted success. I hadn't yet felt the sting.

(No one told me that unless I changed some of my ways, my body would be shot; I would be exhausted, and the money would never be enough.) I found out as I climbed the elusive ladder of success that whatever bad habits I had, or how many thoughts of lack I brought with me on that ladder, I would be carrying it all up with me, rung by rung—on my back, by the way—until I had the courage to let go.

Letting go begins with facing where you are. You can't let go of something until you claim it, know it, embrace it from all sides. Letting go is having the courage to give up dreams that no longer serve you and to look around at reality.

I understand there is a part of you that believes you are in transition, and that when, or *if*, you ever do figure all this out, *then* you will paint the wall, eat healthier, or be open to love. I don't have to tell you how flawed that thinking is. You know it. But still, in some ways, you are hanging on to the wish that maybe, just maybe, some magic will change your life for you. Well, you can sit around and wait, or you can take charge by letting go.

I think it's hard sometimes too face your body image head-on. However, altering your environment can give you the courage to take the steps that seem way too risky.

For instance, the attention you to pay to your external environment tells me plenty about how you're paying attention to your internal health. There is really no difference. If you can't find the motivation to make your bed, do your laundry, or brush your matted dog, how will you ever trust yourself to lose forty pounds, go to the dentist, or take your vitamins? Similarly, if you live inside four nondescript white walls that bore you out of your mind, and you sit or sleep on a generic futon you bought because it was "economical" but makes you feel poor, it's no wonder that your creativity and connection to your self-expression feels like it's going down the toilet. Your inspiration is zilch.

A Colorado Frame of Mind

My search for an ideal external environment brought me to a city that forced me to get in touch with my inner health nut. Three years ago I moved to Boulder, Colorado. I was excited to venture from Los Angeles for a while because Boulder is known for its active lifestyle and clean living, and I needed both. I knew instinctively that the surroundings would force me to become healthier, which has proven to be true. The mind-set there is just totally different.

To start with, getting together with friends in Los Angeles usually includes shopping and lunch, while in Colorado, we meet to hike, bike, or walk. After spending four months a year, on average, in the mountain town, I wasn't sure I'd ever be able to move back to the City of Angels. The thought of reverting to my old walking-up-the-escalator exercise regime scared me. Now that I'm back in Los Angeles taping *Starting Over*, I have found a way to support myself without undoing all the good that Colorado has brought me—I consciously bring that Colorado frame of mind and attitude with me.

Just what is a Colorado attitude? There are three words I would use to describe the lifestyle I embraced in the Rocky Mountain state. *Relax, Rejuvenate,* and *Risk.*

Relax. I wake up in the morning and breathe in the clean, crisp air. I eat a little breakfast as I look at the stunning landscape. I take my time when I'm driving down the mountainous freeways. There's just an ease in my day that I've never experienced before. No stress to get it all done "now." Naturally, as if by a miracle, there's enough time to do everything I've got on my lists, even though I'm multitasking with both hands. The in-between moments aren't filled with worry, stress, or anxiety. Instead, I'm stretching wide and reaching upward. With the mountains looming on the horizon and horses grazing in the pasture beside my home, it's difficult to think anything is more important than right now. The scenery alone makes me stop and take a second look. Forget trying to smell the roses—I can smell 14,000-foot mountains, 100-foot pines, and acres upon acres of wildflowers. I slow down because I don't want to miss the sounds of the bubbling creek, or the aroma of freshly cut hay, or the pitter-patter of a soft spring rain as it cascades down my windowpanes.

Rejuvenate. I walk through town, drinking fresh fruit juice from a local café. I smile and say hello to townspeople I've come to know and love. I laugh as children race through the street on their bikes, heading off for their day's adventures. One of my best friends, Faith, and I meet for our weekly five-mile hike. Taking this time with each other, in nature, has become a higher priority to me than finishing the impossible schedule I had set for myself this week . . . heck, *for the past ten years*! In fact, I'm tired of keeping up with myself anymore, or having to compete with my past performance. I just want to be *me*. The slowed-down, nurturing, more-mellow Rhonda. That means finding the right dosage of regular walks, weekly hikes, and massages that will keep me fit, healthy, nurtured, and strong—whether I think I need them or not. And time—quality time with friends.

Risk. Colorado attracts adventurous spirits. With so many physical activities to participate in, and such beauty in which to do them, it's hard to sit on the couch munching on Pringles. The fresh air and blue sky beckon me outdoors, inviting me to hike to Longs

Peak, ride the white-water rapids down the Colorado River, learn to rock climb, or cycle some of the hundreds of miles of bike trails. You simply can't say no. Even if you've always considered yourself a bit timid or even wimpy, just being around all of these sport-minded people will make you more courageous. Not only did moving to Colorado get me serious about becoming healthy, but I became determined to break the image I had of myself as someone who couldn't hack the wilds. Colorado—the people, the atmosphere, and the weather—had awakened my inner jock, the one who was lying dormant, just waiting to kick some butt and run for the hills, literally, for the first time since high school.

Paying attention to my body only happened when I decided it was worth listening to. That decision came from my commitment to care for myself at a deeper level. I am one of those people who seems to do everything herself. I am self-sufficient, independent, and resourceful. Yet, with all my accomplishments and accolades, I have not been very good at preventing myself from burning out, stressing out, and freaking out. That's where the Colorado frame of mind comes in, the ability to relax, rejuvenate, and risk—because really, if you run yourself into the ground or become stuck in a rut, you can't very well be of any good to anyone else.

Marta was the first one who commented on my change. She noticed that I wasn't so intense, but rather more at ease if things didn't work out just right. She mentioned that I had suddenly quit trying to be perfect, and it seemed that being "important" didn't matter anymore. She wondered if I had acquired more patience because I had been practicing patience with myself.

Then my friend Linda noticed that I was more relaxed when we got together. Our lunches were longer, I laughed about things and situations that used to make me tense, and we had more fun. I was finally creating an environment that was supporting me. The difference in my stress and denial levels was noticeable. Both had substantially decreased.

When you take care of your inner and outer environment, you discover new aspects of yourself that seemed impossible just weeks, days, or even moments before. Colorado gave me the gift of experiencing freedom within my body, something that I didn't know was possible.

I'm not advocating that the entire population of the United States relocate to Colorado. It's not a place as much as it is a state of mind. That's why travel can be so powerful. If you really absorb the essence of each area and what it has to teach you, you can change while you're there and take the lesson home with you. Your Colorado attitude might live with you in Manhattan or the plains of Nebraska or on the Puget Sound. Only you know what calls to your soul, and just because Colorado is my spot, doesn't mean it'll be yours. Everyone is turned on, so to speak, by different environments. Tall trees or tall buildings? Wide open spaces or wide open malls? What ignites my passion may turn you off, and vice versa. That's okay. Each of us must create an environment that nurtures our bodies as well as our souls. And, when you create it with your health in mind, you are automatically supporting any other goals you might have, whether you want to make more money, fall in love, or just have more fun. When you treat your body right, you have a much better chance that it will be right there for you when you need it.

Start Small

Make your personal space more, well, personal. Whether I am living in Los Angeles in a rented apartment or spread out and living large in a big renovated barn in Colorado, I take my collections of rocks, leaves, and beach glass with me everywhere I go. Placing them on my coffee table—any coffee table—signals to me that I'm "home." Another thing that anchors me to home is photos of my sisters, nieces, and nephews, so I make sure to spread those around in an abundant supply.

What makes you feel like you're at home? Maybe it's simply a pillow you have carried around with you since college, or the bear your mother made you for your tenth Christmas, or maybe pulling out a Scrabble board centers you immediately and reminds you of happy times and loved ones.

The more stressed out you are, the more denial you will have in your life, about your life. So stop for a minute. What is your favorite color—the color that makes you happiest when you see it? Green? Yellow? Magenta? Great. Now go paint the wall behind the sofa, or the frame around the mirror, or race out and get that color for your drapes, your bed sheets, or a pillow for your office chair. If you like leaves, put some in a basket on your coffee table like I do. Do you like toy trains? Fabulous. Set one up in your living room or study, and who cares if it doesn't go with the décor? Some people love the little white sparkly lights that light up Christmas trees. Hang some from your window or wrap them around your porch. Feeling good about where you live and the space you create at work is vital to your ability to take more risks in other areas of your life.

If you feel silly or even shameful when thinking about the environment you create for your body, you aren't alone—I promise you.

Most of us don't see the correlation between the inner and the outer, or between our homes and ourselves. But I hope I've shown you, even in a small way, that your surroundings give you subconscious cues. By adding ease, comfort, and safety into our lives through the visual stimulation that plays out in our environments, we're immediately adding to our sense of self and increasing our self-confidence. Claiming your surroundings lets you know that you are taking charge of your life.

Even if you're not able to choose where you work or live right now, due to financial constraints, family obligations, or health challenges, there are other ways you can and do influence your environment. What you read, what you watch on TV, where you sleep, the friends you surround yourself with, all make up your environment, along with your decorating talents, the shoes you wear, and the career you have. Bottom line: Everything you do contributes to your environment, and that environment contributes to your overall sense of accomplishment and overall sense of self, including how you feel about your body.

Your Exercise

I urge you to do the following. For the next week, I want you to rigorously pay attention to your surroundings. Do you feel annoyed as you grab the broken doorknob to the bathroom door or cabinet? Do you get immediately tense when you sit down and face your computer? Do you find yourself saying, "What does it matter?" as you throw your mismatched bedspread on top of your unused treadmill before you hit the hay?

Ask yourself, and write down, what you use as an excuse in your environment to sit at a messy desk, light up that cigarette, or grab that bag of chips. What are you saying to yourself that gives you permission to forget that you matter?

Denise was the wild redhead in the *Starting Over* house with the kind-hearted husband, the woman who absolutely refused to keep her house clean, even at the risk of losing the only man who ever really treated her with care. Denise used any reason she could to stop washing the dishes, not pick up the towels she had thrown on the bathroom floor, or take any kind of grown-up responsibility for her surroundings.

Denise was stuck in what I call "angry child mode," and she wanted someone to save her. But no one would or could, and no one is going to save you either. As Denise learned to clean up her environment, she learned that what the world saw as her outside chaos was really created by her internal chaos. That was a painful lesson, but as she began to understand the symbolism of cleaning up her outer world, she took charge of making her bed, emptying the trash, and hanging up her clothes rather than throwing them in a mound. It didn't take long for her thinking to become clearer. When Denise had a structure in place for cleaning up her house, she had the courage and the energy to clean up her emotions, her marriage, and her life.

As you walk through your home and workplace today, I want you to list the things you see that put a smile on your face. What are you proud of? What looks good to you? What do you want more of? And conversely, what brings down your energy, or even embarrasses you? If someone you loved and respected were coming to see you for the first time, what things would you change, assuming you could, before they walked through the door? Now commit to changing at least one thing that will have an impact on how you view your life. Then make a list of the others—a goal list—and know that in time, you will accomplish them one by one . . . or move already!

Changing the lightbulb that's been burned out for a week might seem like a hassle when you are doing it, but in the end, you will receive more light in your life. Isn't that what we all want?

Daily Living

Now that you are willing to get your house in order, one step at a time, I want you to consider applying that same principle to yourself. What do you need in your life to create less stress?

I have learned that I may not have the time or the money to schedule a month at the beach for some meaningful downtime, but that doesn't mean I can't create pockets of happiness throughout my day. In the beginning it was hard to do (remember my legacy of struggle?) but I was committed to figuring out how to lessen my stress for my health's sake.

What did I learn to do? I have learned to pamper myself throughout the day. I've realized it has to be integrated into my daily schedule or I just won't do it. As I mentioned in Chapter Ten, I get worried about looking like a diva, but really, you have to buck the system and ask for what you want—otherwise, you just won't get it. And let's face it, if you try to do everything yourself, you'll be exhausted and unable to help anyone—*including yourself.*

When it comes to taking care of you, you have to get over your fear of being liked. You have to love yourself more than how much you want others to love you. In a healthy way, I am asking you to consider your needs as important as anyone else's. Let's stop here and contemplate what I'm asking you to do. I'm asking you to choose you. Period.

So are you ready to put yourself first? Let me make it easy. I understand asking for the world may not be appropriate until you build up your "asking" muscle, but you have to start somewhere. . . .

I have realized it is the little things throughout the day that make my day. For example, I like drinking through straws. Scratch that. I *love* drinking through straws. Are they available everywhere I go? No. So instead of complaining about it, I have learned to stuff some in my purse, my car, and in my office. And because my sisters aren't "straw gals," I have had to remind them to pick some up at the store before I come to visit. (I was afraid they would consider me high-maintenance, a pain, but they haven't said a word.) The same thing goes at restaurants. I ask for a straw with my water. Sometimes I get a peculiar look, but who cares? I like straws. They put a smile on my face and make me feel good. What's wrong with that?

Learning to take care of yourself is a process. Most of us don't wake up one day and know how to do it. For me, it took many days of feeling overworked, overstressed, and overwhelmed to take an honest look at my life and ask myself: *How can I bring the Colorado attitude into my daily life?* I had to be truthful and creative. I remember thinking, *If I'm going to keep this up, and continue helping so many women, then I'd better take care of myself.* Taking care of me meant asking for help, asking for what I want, and getting my needs met on the simplest level.

I sat down and did a personal inventory—asking myself what I would need in order to do my work to the best of my abilities and have a better life working twelve to fifteen hours a day. I decided the skill I practiced with the waiters in my life would now come to good use at work. Risk: I handed my boss a list of requests that would rejuvenate me and allow me to relax a little more throughout the day, and you know what? They looked at my requests of straws, a lighted makeup mirror, a ceramic curling iron, makeup sponges, cotton balls, and Q-tips, and didn't blink an eye! My fear was all in my mind! I couldn't believe how easy it was. So, I went back and asked for an electric teapot and got that too! (But don't you worry; I didn't go crazy . . . I brought my own teacups and tea bags.)

Life is about the little moments. I'm so much happier with the little things taken care of that I decided to go one step further and hire myself a personal assistant this year. I've had business support in the past, but no one to do my personal grunt work (for things like running errands, doing the grocery shopping, and so on). I'm telling you, when you're used to doing everything yourself, it's hard to delegate things you think you "should" do yourself. At first I still did my laundry and grocery shopping, until I asked myself, "Then why do I have a personal assistant if I'm going to do all my personal tasks?" The answer was because I felt guilty.

The number one benefit of having help is that I can do more of the work I am meant to do. But more importantly, I can rest. When I have downtime, I can stop and sit. I was sitting in my chair the other day and my assistant walked by on the way to the laundry room. I had a twinge of guilt. *Should I get up and help?* I thought. *I shouldn't just sit here and drink tea when she is working so hard.* And that's when it hit me. The real reason I hired her was to help me maintain the Colorado attitude of relaxation, rejuvenation, and risk in my everyday life. So instead of jumping up like I normally would and being a team player, I just sat there looking out the window at the leaves falling from the trees and didn't move a muscle.

When she walked by again on the way back from the laundry room to my office, I smiled at her and said, "Thank you for being so caring that I am learning how to care for myself." She smiled back, handing me a bottle of Smart Water and told me to drink some.

I leaned my head back, shut my eyes, and was silently thankful for the moment of bliss.

I've learned during my journey of body care that bliss is found in the moments you are willing to be vulnerable and allow yourself to love and be loved. It's kind of like drinking with straws. Drinking out of straws is a way to take care of myself because *I like it*. I know now that I don't have to have any better reason for doing something other than the fact that I LIKE it. I recently did something else that's had a huge effect on my happiness as well—as much as having the assistant or receiving the "extras" from work. Now, don't laugh, because this gives me a bit of bliss every night before I lay me down to sleep. I put an electric teapot in my bedroom, right by my bed! That may not sound like much to you, but it's been heaven for me.

I've always been a tea person, and I love having a cup or two of chamomile tea before bed. For years, I'd drink my tea and then have to get out of bed, put my robe on, go down to the kitchen, and make another cup—which defeated the whole purpose of relaxing in the first place. I never wanted to get out of bed. I wanted to get a good night's sleep. Now, all of that has changed by simply moving the teapot to my bedroom—within arm's reach. I turn on the teapot by my bed; I wash my face, and when I hear that whistle blow, I pop a tea bag in my favorite mug, allowing the water to seep while I hop in the shower. By the time I get out, the tea is perfect. I get into bed to read a great book with a refill at arm's length.

Another way I de-stress my life is to make sure I have plenty of "support tools" around. So, next to my bed, I've placed my journal, my favorite books and magazines, and a basket filled with pens, Post-its, and dark chocolate—in case I want to have a bite with my tea. These may not be the things that would excite you, but how can you make your own day? You don't have to change your whole life. It could be as simple as moving something closer by three feet! Making your own day might be buying six-dollar drawer organizers that separate your eyeliners and mascaras and eye shadows from your lip liners, Chapsticks, and gloss. Do whatever it is that you like. Who cares if people say, "You have a teapot in your bedroom?" "Yep. Sure do." If your friends aren't happy about it, then they're not your friends.

Sometimes the simple things take twenty minutes. I ask you: Are you worth twenty minutes? Are you worth the effort of changing your life by changing one thing in your home environment today to make your life a bit easier? Are you? I guess it comes down to this: Are you up for the challenge?

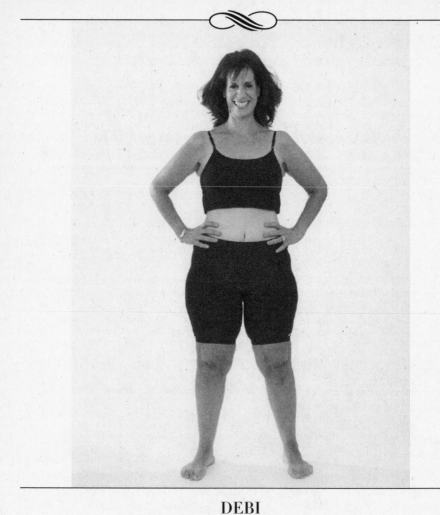

DEBI

Height: 5'5" • Weight: ? • Age: 43

Body Truth: *I'm beginning to love myself and my body, but it's taken thirty years to get here!*

CHAPTER 13

How Can I Get Over
My Body . . . And On
with My Life?

Three years ago I committed to being healthy above all else. I moved to Colorado and gave up dieting for good. No more restrictions. No more deprivation. No more doing whatever it takes to get a great body. No more three months on, three months off. No more trying one diet with no results, then skipping to a new one. No more going to the gym because I was supposed to. No more doing any sort of exercise that I didn't enjoy. No more waking up feeling fat, looking in the mirror, and despising what I saw. In reality, it wasn't working anyway. The strategies I was using to whittle down my waist and lower the number on the scale were ineffective. I can see now that I had the wrong intention all along.

Three years ago, I realized, with sadness and regret, that I may never get my dream body. It was hard to admit, but something I had to face if I was ever going to accept the body I had and really love and make peace with who I was.

When I let go of my fantasy of achieving the "perfect" body, I had to mourn the "loss" of being five feet six inches with a twenty-six-inch waist, firm and toned legs, and rock-hard abs. I had to give up the expectations I had that one day—by some miracle—I would finally have the body of my dreams and my problems would all be solved. Instead, I had to face the fact that my waist wasn't small and hadn't been for years, and that my stomach had never been rock-hard, not *ever*. It was painful to give up the dream because I wanted a different body, a better body, a sexier, more confident, turn-on-the-world body. That body would make me feel powerful. When I finally admitted this desire to myself, I was able to begin the process of surrendering who I thought I *should* be and instead embrace who I was *capable* of becoming.

I was capable of being healthy, and I decided that's what I wanted. Other than some heart palpitations and migraines, there were no medical conditions preventing me from doing more and eating less—not to obtain *"the"* body, but rather to live healthfully in *my* body.

When my motivation changed from "body perfect" to "body healthy," something shifted inside of me. I quit chasing an illusion. I know it might sound like giving up, but in fact, this was the beginning of true freedom for me.

When lifelong health became my commitment, I began to filter all my actions, all my thoughts, all my feelings through that one intention. Going to the bank? I'd ask myself if I could walk instead of drive. What about eating out? I easily altered my choice of restaurants. Making my daily schedule? If self-nurturing and self-care are part of a healthy lifestyle, then massage, downtime, and fun are just as important as finishing up late-night e-mails or deciding whether to attend a meeting or not.

Beginning to live a healthy lifestyle changed my life from the inside out. And that is the miracle. I quit focusing on my measurements, the scale, and calorie counting, and instead began to focus on moving my body for the sake of enjoyment, eating more vegetables because it felt good, and resting a heck of a lot more. I am a recovering workaholic, and like all workaholics, I am vigilant in my choices. Choosing health gave me the focus I needed to change my life.

Getting Over My Body

Three years is a long time to wait for my body to catch up with my healthy lifestyle changes. But that is just what happened. Now, after three years of dedicating my life to health, I am finally seeing, and more importantly *feeling*, the results. And people are noticing.

Men are flirting with me in record numbers. I am being asked out by men fifteen years my junior. My nephews no longer drag me along on vacations; instead, I drag them white-water rafting, rock climbing, and all-terrain-vehicle riding. My nieces, who never exercised a day in their lives, are now joining in. Not only has Deena learned how to cook with health in mind, she is weight training, running, and hiking. Rachel, on the other hand, has joined Pilates and yoga classes while bragging about giving up Pop-Tarts and bagels. Like I shared before, even my sister Linda has gotten into the act. Her extra bedroom is now a mini-gym, with a treadmill and weights strewn about. Cindy, the only sister who has been dedicated to exercise her entire life, is now joining the healthy-food wagon. On our late-night phone calls we discuss our vegetable intake and what aches and pains we're fighting off on our path to health. It feels good. No, wait, that's not true. It feels great!

Millee Taggart-Radcliffe, the executive producer of *Starting Over*, commented on my body just the other day. "Rhonda," she said, "the structure of your body has completely changed. You look so different from Season One." And she's right. Not only do I look different, I *feel* different. I feel beautiful.

It makes me weep. There are almost no words to describe the journey I have been on the past three years. This book has been my attempt at outlining what I did to get from there to here. Yet, words alone aren't enough. Unless you are doing it, committing to it, living it, everything you have read will have little effect on your life. You must do what I say rather than just read about what I did.

I know you want immediate results for your efforts, just like me. But our body doesn't work that way. Our body needs time to heal, to adjust, and to ultimately transform. But we don't give it more than a month here or there. We look for results, and when we don't get them, we move on, never realizing that we were forcing our body to adjust to a foreign way of eating, sleeping, or exercising that may or may not work for us. New habits require a process, and usually aren't noticeable immediately. We forget that change takes time, because we have come to believe that we don't have the time.

In reality, time is all we have. And how you spend your time determines your life.

As I shared with you previously, my weight has only recently started to slip downward. I can finally hear my hunger signals and decipher my cravings, but I must remind myself that it didn't happen overnight. I have been listening to my body intently for over three years.

How did I do it? If you'll remember, I took it slow. By committing to focus my attention on one aspect of my health and make only one major change per year, I figured that the changes would be more permanent. Let's face it, I don't do *anything* slowly, but I knew that if I wanted health above all else, I would have to change the way I treated my body, and therefore, my self. Patience became my middle name. Self-care became my motto. Nurturing my humanity became my number one goal.

Dedicating myself to living a healthy lifestyle day in and day out without any guarantee of results was frightening. There were days I wanted to quit, convinced that what I was doing wasn't working. Even though weight loss wasn't my goal, I secretly prayed the pounds would melt off—and when they didn't, after months of working out and eating "right," I was defeated all over again. When my body didn't respond to my efforts, I assumed that maybe it was too late for me. Maybe I had abused my body so much, and for so long, that it was now unable to respond. But that wasn't true. All my body needed was time. I realize now that time is usually the one thing we refuse to give ourselves.

What did I do the past three years? In the first year I started taking vitamin supplements while upping my vegetable intake and increasing my water intake. Two years ago I started weight training and slowly added cardiovascular workouts, such as getting on my bike and riding for pleasure, hiking, walking with friends, and attending the occasional spinning class. One year ago, I started to focus more on my food choices, which included becoming aware of the foods my body craved, while eliminating the foods that do not serve my health (but almost always served my body hatred). And, throughout the three years, of course I acknowledged my progress and all of my hard work, which gave me consistent support in appreciating my individual process. And, I can't forget my friends who were cheering me along the way.

Sure, I could have done it all at once. That would have been my previous way of doing things, but it never worked in the long run. I could never keep up. The habits never became ingrained; instead I was watching the scale, chasing the dream, and feeling hopeless day after day.

I admit that the old Rhonda would have tried to take off the pounds for the sheer fact that I was on television. I had every reason in the world to get skinny fast. But I had tried that route before and, as I've shared with you, it doesn't work. Not really. Instead, I choose to trust myself, even if people were calling me heavy all over the chat boards. In shutting out their voices and concentrating on what I needed, I faced one of my greatest fears—which ironically is what led me to realizing my goal.

It's not always easy to see the courage in your own actions as it is for a friend or loved one to see them within you. But with my friends' support, I was able to recognize when I had been working hard, regardless of the results (or lack thereof). The changes I made have a much stronger chance of lasting because they were created and built over time. They have become part of the fabric of my everyday experience. They are my daily rituals. I encourage you to follow my lead and see the same future success for your own life.

I understand that three years seems like a long time, but when I put it in the perspective of my whole life and compare it to all the years I spent yo-yo dieting and frantically exercising, three years isn't long at all. The changes I made have been worth the wait. In all honesty, I have wanted to feel and look like I do today for the past fifteen years, and it's always felt out of reach. Not anymore. And in fact, nothing does. Because when I started loving my body, I started loving myself. And nothing feels impossible.

Remember Bethany and her path of self-hatred? Well, after she took responsibility for what she had been doing, she wanted to walk the Path of Self-Love, and just like the Path of Self-Hatred, the Path of Self-Love had markers, too. The markers on the Path of Self-Love that Bethany had to decide to claim for herself were I WILL BE OPEN, ACCEPT SELF, TAKE RISKS, and LIVE FEARLESSLY. Those were the markers for ultimate health that Bethany had to choose to live by if she was ever going to love herself. Was it going to be easy? Not necessarily. Would it be worth it? Absolutely!

What about you? What are the markers you need to accomplish in order to feel satisfied with not only your body, but with yourself? It might mean BEING LIGHTHEARTED or MOVING MY BODY THIRTY MINUTES A DAY or ACCEPTING COMPLIMENTS. When you choose your markers, you are choosing how you will live your life. Choose wisely. You only get one body.

Your Exercise

It's time to recognize the progress you've made in your life. Pick up a pen and piece of paper, and record the significant health markers you've created in your life, and/or those you plan on reaching in your life. What are you willing to do to exercise, to learn to love your body?

Getting On with My Life

Which brings me to where I am today. Three years ago I could barely run a block, let alone a mile. I always had a secret wish of becoming a runner, but with bad hips and memories of shin splints from high school track, it was a dream I had put on the back burner—*for another lifetime*. And anyway, I was a sprinter, so I could just forget about ever belonging to the long, lean running club that flocks to the trails around my home in Colorado like birds to nectar.

And then something happened. My niece Deena moved in with me, and she was inspired by my daily walks, afternoon vegetable breaks, and weight-lifting regime. She wanted to join in and did, but she wasn't content to just walk around the block—she wanted to run around the town. I told her to go ahead, that I couldn't run with her. *She is more than twenty-five years younger than me*, I told myself, *and I've done my job, I've inspired her; now it's up to her to keep it going. I couldn't possibly keep up.* Since I didn't want to hold her back, we would begin our walks together and always end up arriving home separately—her with a shirt soaked in sweat, and me envious of her ability to move so easily in her body.

As my body was turning the corner on the three-year mark, the changes were noticeable and Deena wasn't convinced that I couldn't run. She called me on it, asking me to admit that I did want to run. That wasn't true, I told her, and I proceeded to give her the list of reasons why I couldn't. She simply said, "That was then, this is now." It gave me pause. Isn't that what I teach? That the past does not dictate the future?

I could no longer deny the changes in my body. I was no longer cringing when I looked in the mirror. I had more energy. My yoga poses were bringing ease to my hips. *What if I could run after all and it was only my thinking that was getting in my way?*

With Deena's support, I started by running a block, and then walking the next block. Sure, she still finished way ahead of me, but that didn't seem important anymore. My competitive nature relaxed while a different type of competitive spirit arose within me. Now I was fighting to break the barriers of limitations—my limitations. And I wanted to win.

After three months, I was easily running a mile and feeling stronger and more energetic than I had in years. My success made me want to challenge my body in a big way, a new way. I wanted my mind and my body to become partners in working toward a challenging goal—something that we would have to become totally committed to regardless of our weight, the weather, our moods. Basically, it was time to put my commitment on the line: Was I really willing to become as healthy as I could, or just as healthy as was convenient?

At the checkout stand at my local grocery store, at the bank counter, and in the drug store, I kept seeing signs saying: RUN A MARATHON! WE CAN HELP! My first thought was, *No way. I have no desire. I'm no runner.* But as the signs kept popping up everywhere, "no" turned into "maybe" and eventually into "could I?" *But how?* I thought, *Can I really go from running one mile to running 26.2 miles?* Once again, my dreams seemed impossible.

I laid the brochure next to my bed and every night I stared at it, reading it over and over. It promised a sure, foolproof running plan. It said it was easy, and that anyone could do it. And it kept on inviting me to join them. *Arrgh*, I thought to myself, *what if I fail? What if I can't do it? What if I look like a fool?*

The minute I noticed my line of thinking—that I was worried

about looking foolish—I knew that I had to do it. I knew that fear was trying to run my life, and that was not okay with me! As I tell the women in the *Starting Over* house, any feeling you refuse to feel and face is running your life. I was no fool. I called the marathon help line and said, *"Help!"*

Daniel showed up at my house a week later to test my running ability. I made up lame excuse after lame excuse, making sure he understood that I wasn't a runner and haven't run more than a mile since high school.

He smiled, nodded, and said he understood. *Good*, I thought, *maybe we can run the mile and be done with it. He will tell me I am not ready to run a marathon and this whole thing can be over.*

And with that, Daniel glanced down at his watch, set his timer, and said, "Are you ready?" And we were off. I was panting like a dog in heat by the end of my block, but he kept giving me words of encouragement. So, desperate for approval, I just kept my feet moving, one forward step after another.

Block after block, I kept focused on the next street, the next sign, my house in the distance. *If I can just get to my house*, I thought, *everything will be all right and I will put this charade behind me.*

We were just about at my block when Daniel—who wasn't even breathing hard, I want you to know—warned me that we would not be going down my street. I looked up at him with the biggest doe eyes I could muster, trying not to heave, and prayed that he would change his mind. He ignored me and kept on running. "Inconsiderate male," I muttered quietly. *He isn't even caring about my health right now; he isn't even paying attention to my capabilities. This is clearly dangerous, and more than a mile, I'm sure.* Truth be told, I was worried about how I felt, but even more so about how I must *look. I must look beyond exhausted*, I thought. *Like something the cat dragged in. And aren't I paying for this? Ugh. This isn't fair.*

Daniel interrupted my inner complaining session, declaring that if I could make it to the stoplight ahead I would have run a total of .8 miles. "Point eight miles?" I said, barely able to catch my breath. "You have got to be kidding me. Are you for real? Haven't I run a mile yet?"

Daniel gently assured me that, yes, at the stoplight, .8 miles would be mine, like that was some big accomplishment—the Holy Grail of a runner's first day out. I felt completely deflated, unable to believe that I hadn't run a mile yet. I know I told him I wasn't sure I could, but my competitive nature was getting the best of me. I had run a mile in the past and I was going to show this cocky guy that I could run it again. As I was mulling this around in my head, he started humming the theme song from *Rocky*. *Nice touch*, I thought, as my heavy panting became heavier (and louder) and my breathing more labored.

At this point, my feet were almost numb, and my legs felt like they were about to give up. Falling down then would have been easier than staying the course, but I can be stubborn. So as we reached the stoplight, I announced that I was going to keep going . . . I was going to run a mile if it killed me. *And it just might*, I thought.

As I stumbled to get the words out and keep going, he started laughing. "What's so funny?" I wondered.

"Stop, Rhonda," Daniel ordered, almost on cue. His voice was loud and authoritative, and I wondered if I was about to be reprimanded on that very spot. Secretly thankful that he made me stop, I leaned over and grabbed my legs, trying to catch my breath when he casually announced . . .

"Congratulations. You just ran three miles."

My words came tumbling out faster than my legs had just been running.

"What? I ran three miles? Are you teasing me? Are you sure? I mean, I thought I had run more than a mile, but I didn't know for sure. Are you kidding me? Tell me the truth? Three miles. Wow! Are you sure?"

Daniel assured me that it was all true. I felt on top of the world. I felt like I could do anything. And in some ways, I had done the impossible. I hadn't run three miles since the eleventh grade, more than twenty-five years ago.

I was hooked.

Start Slow and Finish First

The challenge with judging people is that at some point you usually want to join their club. I had thought runners were crazy, waking up at dawn to run while the dew was still on the grass and the birds were still sound asleep. So when I decided to join the pack, it was the answer to a wake-up call that I had been denying for years. I had wanted more health, more vitality, more life, but I just didn't know I could get it. Never in a million years did I think that running held any of the answers for me.

Fast-forward to today. I have just finished running twelve miles this afternoon. *Me?* Yes, you read that correctly. I'm now a runner, who clips six, ten, and twelve miles on a regular basis. For the past few months, I have been running three times a week and sometimes more to prepare to run a marathon. That's right. I am going to run 26.2 miles at one time on one day.

By the time you read this, I may have already run my first one.

I don't know if there will be more after that, but I know that running ties into everything I've been working on for the past three years. For instance, a marathon takes months to train for. You have to start slow (just like I did with my health commitment) to be able to build your endurance in order to finish the race. I started with three miles, built up to four, then five and six, and so on. You cannot skip a step or tempt the fates. I had to follow the rules my body set forth or injury would result. That meant I had to learn to listen to every ache, pain, and growl. I have learned the difference between a shin splint and a muscle that's just stretching, growing, moving past its comfort zone. I have learned the difference between the mental chatter telling me to stop at mile three (rather than run to mile four) and the voice inside my head that tells me to keep going, but slow down, in order to best care for myself. I have learned the difference between downing food for comfort and downing food in order to train at my peak.

I have learned that in order to finish fast, you must start slow. This has become my motto—one I had been exemplifying but wasn't consciously aware of until beginning the long trek to becoming a marathoner.

A marathon is a race I will never win. And that might be the best thing about it. With every mile comes the constant opportunity to face my limitations and my past patterns of defeat. I do want to stop every time I hit mile two. Every single time I pass the three-mile marker, I think I'm crazy and want to give up. But what I have noticed is that if I just stick to it and keep going, mile four is a breeze, just like choosing vegetables over fried foods, or a kiwi over pie.

Change is hard. Our bodies want to heal, but they fight against the discipline needed. So we quit all too soon, convinced that we've been defeated or will never get the results we want, or when we don't feel like it anymore because it's too hard. What I know now is that mile two is hard; mile ten is easy. Life is the same. That is why it can take up to three years for your body to shift into one you can live with. That's why it might take you three years to accept your body as it is, with or without your stomach disappearing.

In order to get over your body and on with your life, you must face the ultimate test: You must decide between you and your fears. That's all it boils down to.

Your fears want to stay safe and stay home when the world looks scary.

In reality, we are all running a marathon. Except crossing the finish line isn't about running 26.2 miles. It's about learning to accept your body as it is; doing what you can to nurture yourself, and most importantly, learning to love all of you, *body and all*.

Ahead of you will be many mile markers. One might read EAT MORE VEGETABLES while another might read WALK A BLOCK or YOU ARE WORTHY. It's up to you to determine the race ahead, and choose the best path for you because, ultimately, you are the one who must live in your body and experience your life. No one can do that for you.

So what do you choose? Choose you!

ABSolution: The Practical Solution for Building Your Best Abs by
Shawn Phillips and Bill Phillips
Body Wars: Making Peace with Women's Bodies: An Activist's Guide
by Margo Maine, Ph.D.
Chris Carmichael's Food for Fitness: Eat Right to Train Right by
Chris Carmichael
*Coming to Our Senses: Healing Ourselves and the World through
Mindfulness* by Jon Kabat-Zinn
*Eat to Live: The Revolutionary Formula for Fast and Sustained
Weight Loss* by Joel Fuhrman, M.D.
The End of Diets: Healing Emotional Hunger by Dilia De La Alta-
gracia
Fat Land: How Americans Became the Fattest People in the World by
Greg Critser
*Food & Mood: The Complete Guide to Eating Well and Feeling
Your Best* by Elizabeth Somer, M.A., R.D.
*Genetic Nutritioneering: How You Can Modify Inherited Traits and
Live a Longer, Healthier Life* by Jeffrey S. Bland, Ph.D. with
Sara H. Benum, M.A.
How We Eat: Appetite, Culture, and the Psychology of Food by
Leon Rappoport

Low-Fat Living: Turn off the Fat-Makers Turn on the Fat-Burners by Robert K. Cooper, Ph.D. with Leslie L. Cooper

Marathon: The Ultimate Training Guide by Hal Higdon

Overcoming Overeating by Jane R. Hirschmann and Carol H. Munter

The Overfed Head: What if Everything You Know about Weight Loss Is Wrong? by Rob Stevens

Self-Esteem Comes in All Sizes: How to Be Happy and Healthy at Your Natural Weight by Carol A. Johnson, M.A.

Self-Nurture Learning to Care for Yourself as Effectively as You Care for Everyone Else by Alice D. Domar, Ph.D.

Tales from the Scale: Women Weigh in on Thunder Thighs, Cheese Fries and Feeling Good . . . at Any Size by Erin J. Shea

The Little Food Book: You Are What You Eat by Craig Sams

When Food Is Love: Exploring the Relationship between Eating and Intimacy by Geneen Roth

Women's Bodies, Women's Wisdom by Christiane Northrup, M.D.

You: The Owner's Manual by Michael F. Roizen, M.D. and Mehmet C. Oz, M.D.

G R A T I T U D E S

Today, I am grateful for . . .

Linda Sivertsen, my right arm in creating this book. Her editorial guidance, insightful comments, brainstorming, and interviewing support made a good book great.

Mary Ann Halpin. Thank you for sharing your award-winning talent as a photographer by creating a space where each woman was free to express her true feelings about her body.

Maria Akl, story editor. Thank you for taking hours of raw footage and turning it into a moving piece explaining the truth about our relationships with our bodies. Thank you to Joe Croyle and his team for their supreme efforts in capturing the day beautifully.

Brian Tart, president and publisher of Dutton, encouraged me to write this book in the first place. His unfailing support for my work has given me the freedom few writers experience. Neil Gordon, editorial assistant, thank you for your humor and support.

Meg Leder, editor, and Michelle Howry, senior editor, of Perigee Books. WOW! Your detailed commitment to my work inspires and humbles me. Thank you.

Amy Williams, literary agent extraordinaire. Your belief in me makes me better.

Helen Shabason, television agent. Thank you for always being my cheerleader, going to bat for me no matter what and finding humor in impossible situations.

Gordon Corte, Lisa Roina, and Jason Pinyan of ICM. Thanks for spreading my work.

The entire staff at Dutton, thank you! This is our fourth book together and I want to thank you for always watching my back and taking care of business. Double thanks to Kathleen Schmidt for putting my work out into the world and, more importantly, believing in it. And special thanks to the sales team for always going the extra mile.

Jon Murray, Joey Carson, and Millee Taggart-Radcliffe, executive producers of *Starting Over*. Thank you for giving me the gift of sharing my work though the medium of television. I love what I do because of your support, care, and absolute integrity.

Linda Midgett, Adriane Hopper, and Laura Korkoian, supervising producers of *Starting Over*. Thank you for supporting me while writing this book. Your willingness to give me the space, time, and energy to do two major projects at once was a godsend. And a special thank-you to Dr. Stan Katz, who keeps me sane and centered.

The entire production crew of *Starting Over*. Bruce Ready, Dana DeMars, James Lockard, Matt Gatson, and everyone else. How do I thank you for putting your lives on the back burner day in and day out as we change women's lives? You always put the women first. You always want me to look good. You always care about the process. A special shout-out to Jen Klein, who is my angel. Thank you for going above and beyond.

Jeff Zucker, Frederick Huntsberry, Barry Wallach, Linda Finnell, Regina Thomas, and the entire NBC Universal family. Thank you for continuing to put your trust in me and believing in

Starting Over. I love what I do and am honored I've been chosen to do it!

Joe Schlosser, VP of communications at NBC Universal, and your entire team. The *Starting Over in America* tour rocked!!! Thank you for giving me the opportunity to feel like a rock star. Hats off to Todd Beck and Steve Spignese of Beck Media for their hard work!

Beth Karish, executive director of the Fearless Living Institute. There are no words to express my love and appreciation for what you do all day long with such love, such care, and such commitment. You turn my dreams into reality every day. Thank you! I love you! And let's not forget the ever faithful Steven Bartu, office manager. What a gem!

The Fearless Living Institute Core Team and Wise Council, the Certified Fearless Living Coaches who are on the ground spreading the principles of Fearless Living. Jerilyn Thiel, Susie Peterson, Bill Grout, Rosie Laughlin, Kristin Bendixen, Cindy Tvinnereim, Martha Pasternak, Faith Davis, Sandy Goodwin, Wendy Perkins, and Josie Sullivan. Your commitment and love inspire me to be better. Always know I am grateful.

Sarah Hallman, my personal assistant. Thank you! Thank you! Thank you! Your nurturing essence and attention to detail have saved me too many times to mention.

Andy Paige, my ever faithful image consultant. I feel more beautiful because of you. I am grateful.

Angela C. Montano, my spiritual support. Your commitment to spirit living through us and as us continues to ground me in the reality of the divine. Thank you for your prayers.

Cindy, Linda, Deena, and Rachel, and the newest addition, Marcie . . . the women of my family. Our talks about our bodies inspired me and guided me throughout these pages. May you always know how much I love you. And to the men in the family, Dean, Joel, Jason, Adam, and Zachary . . . the five most important men in my life, whom I am honored to know and love.

Family and friends . . . you know who you are . . .

Fearless Living Institute Web site members. You are the courageous ones!

You! Your willingness to face your body and learn to love it lets me know there is a need for this message. I pray that we all learn that we are enough exactly as is and that we have the right to live the life our soul intended. . . .

READY TO BECOME
FEARLESS . . .

Work with a Certified Fearless Living Coach?
Attend a Fearless Foundation workshop?
Lead or join a Fearbuster Group?
Want to become a Life Coach?

To find out more about *Do I Look Fat in This?* workshops and teleclasses, available private Life Coaches trained by Rhonda, all the ins and outs of starting your own Fearbuster Group, opportunities to meet Rhonda in person, and the latest happenings . . .

Visit Rhonda's Web site: www.FearlessLiving.org.

Want to learn at your own pace,
on your own schedule?

Become a paid member of the Fearless Living Institute (FLI) Web site and receive access to hundreds of hours of Rhonda sharing what she knows through audio clips and videos. You will be able to learn in the comfort of your home, on-demand.

Visit Rhonda's Web site: www.FearlessLiving.org.

Become a Certified Fearless Living Coach . . .

The Fearless Living Institute (FLI) has the most thorough, comprehensive, and business-building coaching training program in the world. It is the only coaching program that requires you to complete four prerequisites, helping you find out if becoming a coach is really for you, saving you money and time. For more information, log on to www.FearlessLiving.org.

Would you like your business to be more Fearless . . .

The Fearless Living Institute (FLI) is the gold standard for human potential in the business world! Benefits to our programs designed specifically for you are: higher retention through increased employee and client satisfaction; increased staff productivity; maximum bottom-line efficiency; and a renewed ability to tap into the creativity and ingenuity of your employees. Contact the Fearless Living Institute at (303) 447-2704.

ABOUT THE AUTHOR

Rhonda Britten, named America's Favorite Life Coach, is the founder of the Fearless Living Institute—featuring the world's premiere life- and career-coach training program. As the Life Coach on the Emmy Award–winning daytime reality drama *Starting Over,* she has been called its "Most Valuable Player" by the *New York Times.*

Having developed the leading model for mastering emotional fears, Rhonda has written several national bestsellers based on her fearless principles, including *Change Your Life in 30 Days, Fearless Loving,* and *Fearless Living* (translated into twelve languages).

As a speaker, she wows corporations with her high-impact, right-on message of personal accountability while giving them practical, hands-on tools that make a bottom line difference. Corporate clients have included Southwest Airlines, Northrop Grumman, and Blue Shield.

For more information on Rhonda, visit www.FearlessLiving.org.

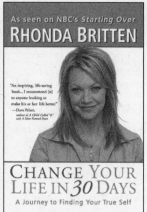
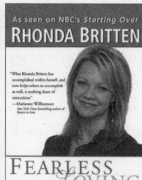
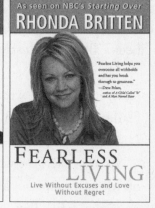